Praise for **Jorge Cruise** and *The Belly Fat Cure*

"Jorge Cruise gets it right by eliminating excessive sugar and processed carbohydrates. His recipes make eating smart easy. I recommend them highly."

— **Andrew Weil, M.D.,**
Director of the Arizona Center for Integrative Medicine,
University of Arizona, and author of *Why Our Health Matters*

"The message is simple: eating fat does not make you fat; rather, eating the right types of fat can help you lose fat. Make a few simple changes to your lifestyle and get on the Fast Track to losing your belly fat today."

— **Terry Grossman, M.D.,**
co-author of *Transcend: Nine Steps to Living Well Forever*

"When it comes to your health, forward thinking will allow you to avoid obesity and disease and achieve longevity. Jorge's program springs from progressive science that can truly change your body—and it all starts with controlling your consumption of sugar and processed carbs."

— **Ray Kurzweil,**
world-renowned scientist and author of *The Singularity Is Near: When Humans Transcend Biology,* and *Fantastic Voyage: Live Long Enough to Live Forever*

"Jorge, again, is on to something; belly fat is surely an indicator of poor health. This book will turn your life around."

— **Suzanne Somers,**
actress, and best-selling author of *Breakthrough: Eight Steps to Wellness*

The

BELLY FAT
CURE™
FAST TRACK

The
BELLY FAT CURE™

FAST TRACK

Discover the **ULTIMATE CARB SWAP**™ and drop up to 14 lbs. the first 14 days

JORGE CRUISE

HAY HOUSE, INC.
Carlsbad, California • New York City
London • Sydney • Johannesburg
Vancouver • Hong Kong • New Delhi

Published and distributed in the United States by: Hay House, Inc.: www.hayhouse.com • *Published and distributed in Australia by:* Hay House Australia Pty. Ltd.: www.hayhouse.com.au • *Published and distributed in the United Kingdom by:* Hay House UK, Ltd.: www.hayhouse.co.uk • *Published and distributed in the Republic of South Africa by:* Hay House SA (Pty), Ltd.: www.hayhouse.co.za • *Distributed in Canada by:* Raincoast Books: www.raincoast.com • *Published in India by:* Hay House Publishers India: www.hayhouse.co.in

All photos and illustrations courtesy of JorgeCruise.com, Inc.

<u>The JorgeCruise.com, Inc., team:</u> *Head writer:* **Evan Dollard**/JorgeCruise.com, Inc. • *Creative editor:* **Michelle McGowen**/JorgeCruise.com, Inc. • *Visual director:* **Jared Davis**/JorgeCruise.com, Inc. • *Managing director:* **Oliver Stephenson**/JorgeCruise.com, Inc. • *Mental-health director:* **Marta Fox**/JorgeCruise.com, Inc. • *Client support:* **Chance Miles and Stephen Steigler**/JorgeCruise.com, Inc. • *Personal assistant:* **Kim Barry**/JorgeCruise.com, Inc.

TRADEMARKS

The Belly Fat Cure	3-Hour Diet	JorgeCruise.com
The BellyFatCure.com	3HourDiet.com	Time-Based Nutrition
Carb Swap System	8 Minutes in the Morning	Tasty Carb Swaps
S/C Value	Super Carbs	Happy Hormones, Slim Belly
Body at Home	Restorative Proteins	Women's Carb Cycling
Ulitmate Carb Swap	Be in Control	Sugar Calories
12-Second Sequence	Controlled Tension	The 100
12Second.com	Jorge Cruise	

Library of Congress Control Number: 2014949726

1st edition ISBN: 978-1-4019-2914-5
Revised edition ISBN: 978-1-4019-4671-5

13 12 11 10 9 8 7 6 5 4
1st edition, September 2011
4th (revised) edition, January 2015

Printed in the United States of America

To Carol Brooks

Contents

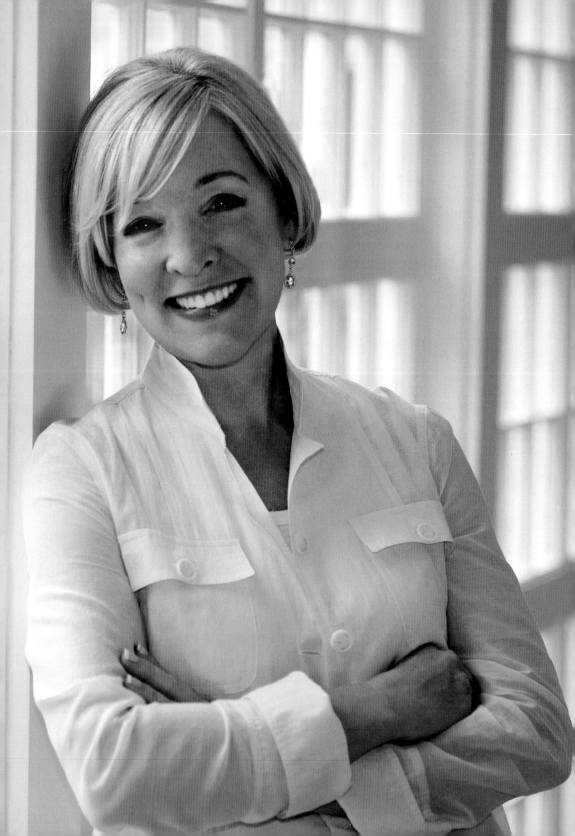

Dear Reader,

Some of my fondest childhood memories are of going out for ice cream on a summer night, or driving with my family to Sherm's Cookie Kitchen. Sherm was an old man who baked delicious cookies and breads and also kept us kids enthralled with his mesmerizing stories. The sweetness of summer, the cookies, and the stories all created a strong link in my mind and body.

But there was a dark side to all of this sweetness. In the 8th grade, I was one of the heaviest in my class. That's why I went on my first diet. Yet it only seemed to lead to another diet and then another, each more difficult than the last. Whether it was macrobiotic vegan, Atkins, or low carb, I've been there. Lurking in the background all those years was always a craving for sugar. I have struggled most of my life to maintain a healthy weight—a struggle that picked up speed at midlife.

Finally I discovered the work of Jorge Cruise, and learned about hidden sugars in foods. I knew about the glycemic index and that too much refined and added sugar wreak havoc on the immune system, but I had never thought about the total sugar content of my daily diet as an absolute. When you start reading labels and see how much sugar is in common foods, you'll be as shocked as I was. The medical literature is finally catching up with the fact that fat is not the problem we've been led to believe it is. It's sugar. Sugar gets turned into fat in the body very, very quickly.

I've sat with thousands of women who have experienced exactly the same lifelong struggle with their weight as I have. As someone who has been on the leading edge of women's health for 30 years, I can assure you that the answer to the weight dilemma—and many of the health conditions that go along with it, such as high blood pressure, diabetes, heart disease, and cancer—lies in decreasing the amount of sugar in your diet from all sources and adding back healthy fats and protein.

I'm eternally grateful to Jorge Cruise for creating a simple lifestyle plan that shows you exactly how to remove excess sugar from your diet, while returning healthy, satisfying fats to their proper place. The Belly Fat Cure works. After all these years, my weight is finally stable, and sugar no longer calls to me from every bakery window I pass. I want the same for you. This book will show you how.

— **Christiane Northrup, M.D.**

Christiane Northrup, M.D., a board-certified ob-gyn, is the *New York Times* best-selling author of *Women's Bodies, Women's Wisdom; The Wisdom of Menopause;* and *The Secret Pleasures of Menopause.* Through her exclusive Women's Wisdom Circle, Dr. Northrup shares cutting-edge medical and lifestyle advice. For more information, go to: **www.DrNorthrup.com.**

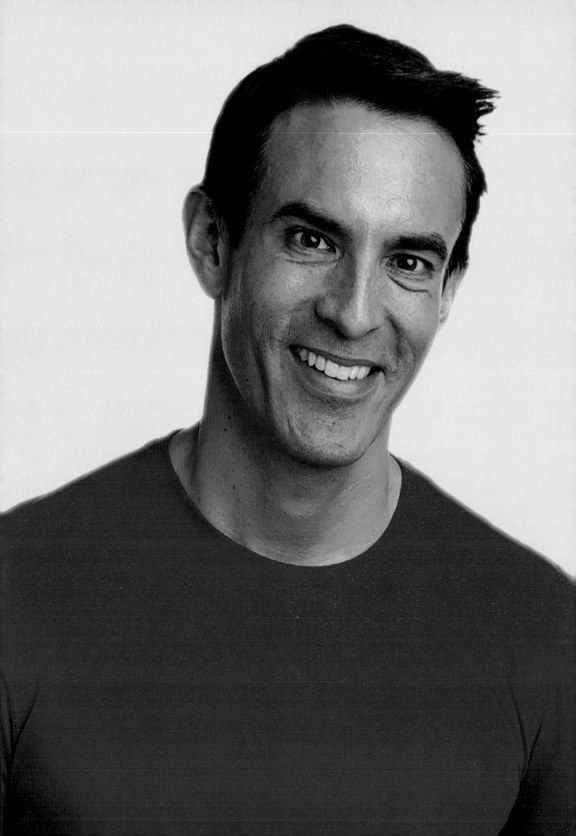

Dear Friend,

Welcome to the Belly Fat Cure revolution! This all-new book builds upon the discovery of my original #1 *New York Times* bestseller, *The Belly Fat Cure:* avoiding hidden sugars—not calories—is the key to true weight loss. Join over a million people who have experienced the transformative power of the original Belly Fat Cure program.

While reading all the exciting success stories on Facebook, many clients asked me, "How can I lose all the belly fat *in less time?"* This book is the answer.

The secret to accelerating belly fat loss is in the power of the Ultimate Carb Swap™. This new tasty and simple strategy will allow you to lose up to 14 pounds in 14 days. And here's the best part: all you need are the everyday foods already in your kitchen or at any local grocery store.

Imagine *enjoying* the foods that melt belly fat and ending each day with a glass of wine or a sweet treat like my famous Chocolate Lace Cookies.

Bon appétit!

Your coach,

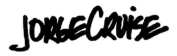

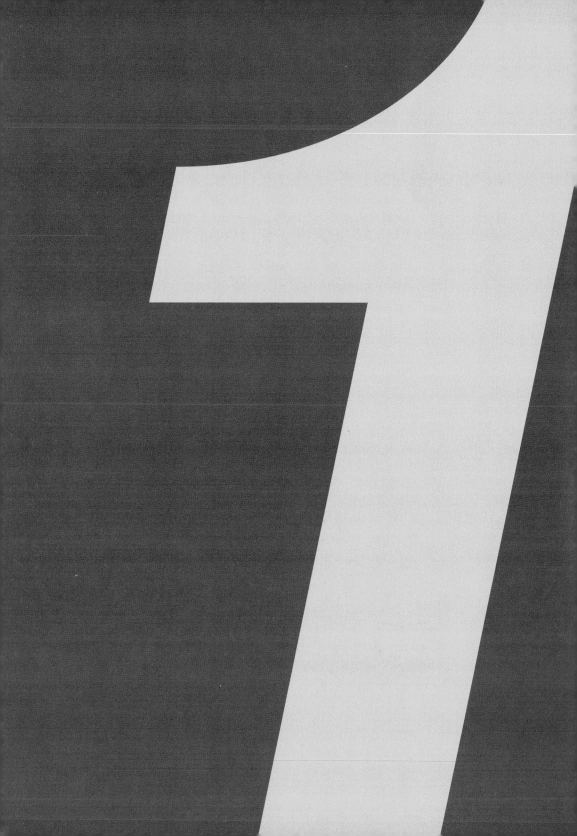

1 14 Pounds
in 14 Days

"You must be the change you wish to see in the world."

— MAHATMA GANDHI

America has reached the breaking point, and yet it continues to barrel forward at a breakneck pace. With such tremendous momentum pushing families and the country toward disease, it is going to take a massive shock in order to correct course and ensure their survival. My hope guides me to believe that *The Belly Fat Cure Fast Track* may provide just such a shock.

Take some time to read the first couple chapters of this book and you will discover the truth about weight loss that

> *Hidden sugar:*
> *The sugar you consume without realizing it, or because you have been led to believe is healthy. Classic examples include milk, fruit, yogurt, bread, juice, and practically every low-calorie or low-fat diet food ever created.*

has been concealed since the beginning of the last century: **hidden sugar** is the true cause of weight gain, not calories. Realizing you have been fed misinformation will free you to finally have the power to control your health and well-being. You will be able to shed up to 14 pounds of belly fat in the first two weeks with my all-new "ultimate" Tasty Carb Swaps exclusive to this Fast Track book. So get ready to look and feel great in all your clothes again!

Just for a moment, consider that almost everything you have been told about what makes us gain weight around our waists has been completely wrong. You do not have to believe that statement just yet . . . you need only *consider* it in order to receive the life-changing value of the information in this book. You may save your final judgment for a very bright morning that awaits you only 14 days from today.

Calories vs. Hidden Sugar

From weight-loss television shows and magazine articles to university research and government recommendations, there are many different groups trying to save the Western world from obesity and disease . . . and just as many conflicting views on the best way to do so. However, my desire is to awaken the planet to the truth about what really causes belly fat: **the foods we eat that are packed full of *hidden* sugar.**

My team and I are certainly the underdogs here, upheld by truth and scientific fact rather than funding and coverage from the conglomerates that profit from your yo-yo dieting and disease.

The latest breakthrough research has proven that losing and gaining belly fat is *not* controlled by how many calories we eat and how many we burn through exercise. That is why the focus of the Belly Fat Cure program has always been to eat the right amount of sugar and carbohydrates to maximize belly fat loss while still satisfying

Insulin:

The regulator of blood sugar, this hormone also drives cells to burn carbohydrates instead of fat and indirectly stimulates the production of more fat. The imbalance of this critical hormone sets off a chain reaction that negatively impacts almost every corner of the body, and is the most profound health crisis facing our modern society.

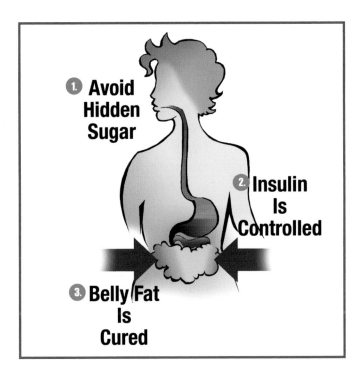

your sweet tooth. The reason we single out sugar and carbohydrates, rather than calories or fat, is linked to the science of the naturally occurring hormone at the center of this program: **insulin.**

Most people have heard of insulin and know that it is something diabetics need to control, but the true nature of this hormone has been poorly communicated to men and women who desperately need the information, with disastrous repercussions. It is with sincere conviction that I will assert the following point throughout this book: the imbalance of insulin in almost all people is the single most deadly, fattening, costly, and misery-inflicting threat to our society at present.

Now, I know what you're thinking: *But I'm not diabetic—my insulin is fine!* or *Of course it's bad to eat sugar, which is why I rarely have candy.* That is where the amazing discovery about insulin and the massive amounts of hidden sugar in our everyday "health" foods comes into play. It is vital to your weight loss that you master the knowledge that **insulin controls not only your blood sugar, but also your body's ability to create and store fat—especially the dangerous fat tissue that accumulates around the midsection.**

Without lowering insulin levels, it is impossible to lose weight, regardless of calorie deprivation or exercise intensity. This explains why some people, if unaware of insulin's role, can feel like they're doing everything right without seeing any results.

Perhaps you are personally familiar with such a scenario, as most of my clients were. However, rather than focusing on the sad story of how this weight loss "silver bullet" has managed to stay covered up for so long—and all the disease that resulted from the cover-up—let us instead look on the bright side.

> **If you control insulin by avoiding hidden sugar,**
> **you will have your foot on the brake pedal**
> **of your body's fat-storage mechanism.**

14 Pounds in 14 Days

How can avoiding hidden sugar help you to lose up to 14 pounds in 14 days? Is it even safe to lose so much weight in such a short period of time? Furthermore, where does that weight come from?

There are perhaps dozens of ways to lose 14 pounds so quickly, even though it may sound like fantasy instead of an achievable goal. Physical exhaustion coupled with starvation seems relatively effective, and sure makes for some great television! Or perhaps bone shaving and a popcorn diet would deliver those same results. Either way, it is certainly possible. The real question at hand is this:

Is it *safe* or *desirable* to lose
up to 14 pounds in 14 days?

The answer is a surprising "Yes!" Now, swimming with sharks can be done safely, as can bungee jumping. The core of each activity, however, remains relatively risky despite whatever precautions are taken. That is not the kind of program I'm delivering to you in this book. You will *not* be engaging in some dangerous weight-loss adventure, comforted by precautionary measures to protect you from injury or death.

It is with this in mind that I reveal not just the only *safe* way to drop up to 14 pounds in 14 days, but also the only truly healing way of making such a drastic transformation in so little time.

Where Does the Weight Come From?

Let me be clear: **it is neither possible nor desirable to lose 14 pounds of *fat* in only two weeks.** The weight lost during the initial transition toward your new body comes from several places, and seeing how all these pieces contribute to your metamorphosis will help you understand how the program works.

Fat: Physiologically, it is only safe to lose about two to three pounds of pure fat in one week without resorting to starvation or dangerously exhaustive exercise. That generally holds true for all people and weight-loss programs, because one pound of fat on your body contains the same amount of energy as a pound of fat on anyone else's body. In today's world, where loud and over-the-top marketing claims are desperately trying to grab your attention, three pounds of pure fat may not sound like a lot, but think of it this way: each pound of fat you lose is like removing four sticks of butter from your body.

Water: Consuming excessive sodium from processed foods can cause swelling and water retention. This bloating is even more noticeable if the diet is also very low in potassium, which is common with overconsumption of sugar, starches, and processed foods. (Although excess sodium from processed foods is harmful, I recommend using sea salt in moderation.) On this program you will avoid processed foods, which can cause bloating and swelling, and you may lose some retained water weight as your sodium and potassium levels become balanced.

False belly fat: Much of the initial weight loss will be the result of reducing the amount of a rather unpopular substance in your own body that I call **false belly fat.** Due to years of dietary devastation, our digestive systems are packed with pounds of trapped waste. I devote all of Chapter 3 to the critical issue of repairing this damage in order to both clean out the system and prepare it to absorb all the rejuvenating nutrients it will soon be receiving.

False belly fat:

Trapped waste matter that adds pounds and inches to the belly, and can also interfere with the absorption of nutrients and healthy digestion.

Cleansing false belly fat over the course of two weeks can cause a significant reduction in real poundage, and contribute to a reduction in waist circumference from bloating and intestinal inflammation. Thus, although bringing balance to your hormones with the Fast Track program comes with a cascade of health and weight-loss benefits, the dramatic weight loss and belly-shrinking results you will experience in the first two weeks are primarily a result of the reduction of false belly fat.

This phenomenon of weight loss from areas other than stored fat is essentially a part of every diet claim in history, but no one has ever seemed to publicize it . . . until now. It is my belief that only when people fully understand the whole truth can they make the best decisions for themselves. I also believe that losing pounds of false belly fat isn't something to cover up, but to celebrate!

I hope all the variables that factor into your numerical weight might also encourage you to do one more thing: pay less attention to your scale! While I know that you will probably continue to weigh yourself at least through the 14 days, please use the information in this section to put your numerical weight in context. Weight seems to tell us many things while actually telling us nothing at all. For this reason, I recommend monitoring the fit of your clothes or measuring your waist to gauge your physical progress on the program. I offer a free how-to video that demonstrates the way to measure your waist on my website: **TheBellyFatCure.com**.

New Information, Accelerated Results

Despite the subtle differences between this book and the original *Belly Fat Cure,* both versions still share the same heart. The Fast Track was created to enhance the original program by offering another avenue for those who want to *accelerate* their health and weight-loss results. It also takes into account that different people can often benefit from different strategies. Many of my successful clients have chosen to alternate between the two programs for long-term success.

Also, 2010 was a great year for breakthrough science that points to a nutritional awakening in our society, and I was incredibly privileged to meet experts who opened my eyes to additional information, foods, and tactics that I wanted to include in this advanced version of the Belly Fat Cure program. Since our world is in a state of constant transition, I promise to continue to seek out the newest information and to make my recommendations for you based on the most current findings.

What Is Unique about the Fast Track?

Here are the key elements that make the Fast Track program different from other weight-loss programs, each of which will be explained in greater detail throughout the rest of the book:

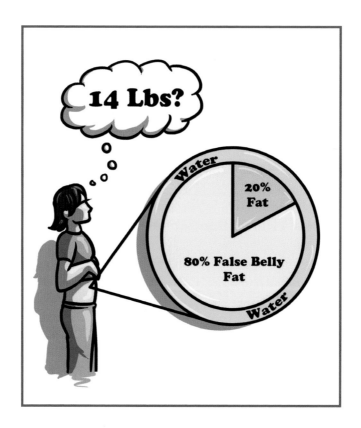

Lose all the weight in half the time! The secret of the Fast Track program combines the strategy of avoiding hidden sugar with the power of the Ultimate Carb Swap to detoxify, banish hunger, and bring balance to your hormones. Working in concert, these two elements can double your weight loss compared to those bland low-fat diets of the past.

Start immediately with foods you can find anywhere . . . even in your own kitchen! The foods that form the foundation of the Fast Track can literally be found at almost any grocery store in the world, and you already have a lot of the key ingredients for success. There are no required specialty foods, no diet foods, and no reason why you can't eat well even if you are traveling. These everyday foods that may already be in your kitchen allow you to start right now!

There is no required tracking or point counting on the Fast Track. You heard me right: no tracking or counting. If you're a fan of the first two books in *The Belly Fat Cure* series, you may be wondering where the S/C (Sugar/Carb) Value fits in. This tool, which helped you uncover and track the tremendous amounts of sugar and carbohydrates lurking in so many products, will still be very useful when you return to the original program. However, you can save time and effort by simply following the Fast Track Menu for 14 days—and then by sticking to the list of what I call Belly Best Foods if you decide to continue with the accelerated program. The beauty of the Fast Track program is that it makes being mindful of sugar and carbohydrates more intuitive by essentially making the S/C Value built in!

More Benefits of the Belly Fat Cure

Since writing *The Belly Fat Cure,* I've discovered a whole host of additional benefits of reducing all forms of sugar in the diet and balancing your hormones. One critical bonus of this lifestyle is that it encourages the production of a very special messenger in your body called *nitric oxide.* Nitric oxide is a gas produced by the lining of your blood vessels and is responsible for their dilation, which decreases your blood pressure and increases blood flow to tissues. This is essential because there is a blood vessel within a micron of each and every cell in your body, and blood is the medium that carries energy and nutrients to your cells. You know that feeling you get when you walk into a stuffy old house? An increase in nitric oxide in your body is like opening every single door and window, allowing fresh air and life to rush into the rooms (the trillions of cells) of your house.

Eating foods free of hidden sugar isn't the only way to sustain levels of what Dr. Christiane Northrup calls "the molecule of the fountain of youth." Happy thoughts, a positive outlook, laughing, and even intimacy are all completely healthy and engaging ways of increasing levels of nitric oxide, and thus increasing the flow of energy and rejuvenation to your entire body. Dr. Northrup points out that each and every one of us was conceived in a burst of nitric oxide, otherwise known as an orgasm, so this molecule's role in our lives cannot be overstated.

The foods I recommend in these pages are also anti-inflammatory. Inflammation is the body's response to a substance it deems harmful, and can be a vital function for healing the body and avoiding infection. However, *chronic* inflammation resulting from a poor diet is a continuous, prolonged response by the body to toxic substances and compounds that it thinks are foreign invaders.

From the perspective of vanity, chronic inflammation can cause swelling and bloating, and is at the root of acne. From the perspective of total health, chronic inflammation has been implicated in numerous ailments including asthma, arthritis, and inflammatory bowel disease. Chronic inflammation also lays the foundation for developing more serious autoimmune disorders.

The Cost of Obesity: One Nation's Case Study

The starring role that **the calorie myth** has been given in the saga of weight loss and optimal health is the primary reason almost 90 percent of Americans are projected to be overweight within our lifetime. Perhaps a country full of overweight, sick citizens doesn't seem too scary to you . . . so long as people are capable of using a keyboard and mouse, they can remain viable parts of the economy, right? Let's try to get a clear perspective of the situation by using a powerful metric that is familiar to most people: *money.*

The calorie myth:

Often referred to as "calories in, calories out," this myth assumes that calorie intake is the only factor involved in successful weight control.

While you are no doubt familiar with money, you are probably not familiar with money in the way I will briefly discuss. According to a study published in the journal *Obesity,* if current trends hold, the U.S. will be spending 18 percent of health-care dollars on obesity and obesity-related diseases by 2030. **The United States of America could end up spending $956 billion per year to manage the complex symptoms of a very simple problem.** Allow me to frame that astronomical figure:

- It is $425 billion more than the budget for the Department of Defense for 2010.

- It is $219 billion more than Medicare and Medicaid combined for 2010.

- It is almost three times the amount spent to pay off the interest of the national debt in 2010.

Given the potentially disastrous economic collapse America (and the world) has been flirting with in recent years, I don't feel that I am in any way being dramatic or apocalyptic when I suggest that such an enormous drain on financial resources con-stitutes a genuine issue of national security. If the ship maintains its current course and the levels of disease and spending reach those projected, the world as we know it may become a very different place.

Gloom and doom have certainly become staples in the current economic and political climate. Because I personally believe in a "glass half full" approach, let's look at those gut-wrenching numbers from a different perspective.

What could the U.S. do with $956 billion a year in savings?

Go ahead, be creative! What could America do? Just remember that this money belongs to everyone: it is the people who work hard to create that wealth. Yet by simply putting the wrong amount of sugar in their mouths, they could throw it all away. Yes, this problem is enormous, but it can be solved . . . and then the *benefits* will be enormous!

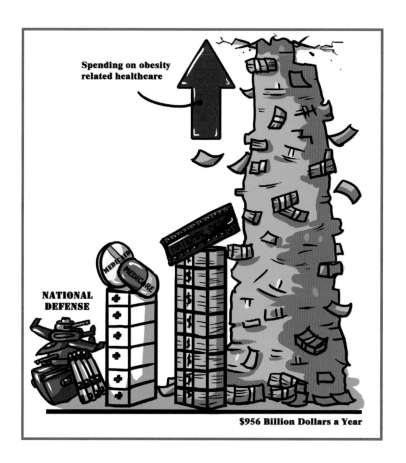

Even better, as I have explained and will continue to reiterate throughout this book, we already know the solution to the problem. My hope is that you will help me in educating America and the world on the simple fix needed to avoid a nightmare scenario in the near future. Ultimately, it would be great to see young people educated more thoroughly on the truth regarding nutrition, disease, and a healthy body weight. In the meantime, what we need is a massive viral campaign to spread the transformative results of this program. **Join the revolution! Start the Belly Fat**

Cure Fast Track program and lead by example to help promote the change worldwide.

Visit **JorgeCruise.com** right now and help me move a few steps closer to my life's goal of changing the way our world eats. Join my e-mail club and take just one minute to share the message with three people you love. You will then have partners along your journey to health, a powerful factor in success that cannot be replicated or overstated. You will become a part of the change you wish to see in the world, and there is hardly a more powerful thing you can do with your time on this planet.

Enter the Fast Track

Whether you are new to the Belly Fat Cure entirely or find yourself on this page to enhance the results you achieved with the original program, it is now time to accelerate your fat loss with the Fast Track program. Many of my clients followed the program for 14 days and lost 14 pounds. Some clients lost more, and others slightly less, but I guarantee *you will* lose belly fat and experience an astounding transformation if you commit to this program for 14 days. For many people, this empowering solution has gone far beyond the first 14 days to become a lifestyle with incredible results. But for now, I advise you to focus on just two short weeks, and get ready to lose belly fat.

FAST TRACK
SUCCESS
STORY

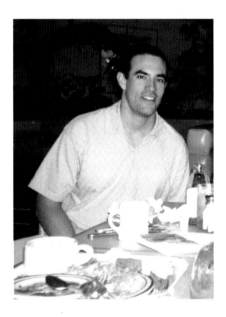

Before

Age: 40

Height: 6'0"

Pounds Lost: 40

Growing up in a poor Mexican-American family, I experienced firsthand the ignorant, Belly Bad eating habits most of us learn in the United States, beginning at a young age. Even worse, as I reached high school I sought more and more comfort in sugary foods to numb the anxiety I felt, and I almost died from a burst appendix. At 40 pounds overweight, I finally discovered the importance of the food I was putting in my mouth. Now, thanks to my Carb Swaps, I am healthier and happier than at any point in my entire life.

I am incredibly blessed to have the opportunities I do, and with these opportunities has come an even greater responsibility. That is why I have devoted the rest of my life to one extremely important mission: to spread the power of my Tasty Carb Swap meals. With your help, I am striving to change the lives of millions of people.

What's Next?

My goal is to change the way the world eats, of course! I have written a lot of books and have met a lot of people, but never before have I been so passionate about my work or about any cause. I am devoting the rest of

Jorge
Lost 40 pounds!

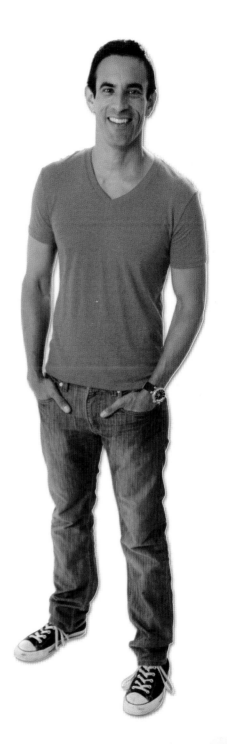

my professional career to spreading the core message of my Carb Swap recipes around the world, because I believe it is critical for future generations that *our* generation learn how to make meals that are yummy, but "Belly Good," too. The habits—and, therefore, the health—that our children and grandchildren will inherit are the habits we have right now. That is why we must be the change we wish to see in the world!

My Best Tip

I fully admit to having a sweet tooth, and keeping it satisfied with smarter options keeps me right on track. By simply knowing in the back of my mind that I can whip up a delicious Fast Track treat whenever I like, I never feel the desire to cheat on the rest of the program. Always having a can of low-sugar whipped cream in my fridge and some dark chocolate handy has been my saving grace!

FAST TRACK
SUCCESS
STORY

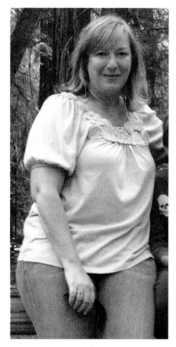

Before

Age: 40
Height: 5'6"
Pounds Lost: 54

Getting dressed for my son's fifth birthday party, I realized that none of my clothes fit me. At first I thought I'd washed everything in hot water by accident, but then the realization set in that it was *me,* not the clothing. I felt helpless and hopeless, knowing I had to lose weight but with no idea how to do so. Somehow I knew that sugar was part of the problem and made a doctor's appointment, expecting to be told that I was prediabetic. At the same time that my test results came back (all good), I found Jorge's plan, and it addressed exactly what I needed.

During Week 4, everything clicked for me, and I knew this was really going to work. It wasn't a gimmick or a fad; it was a real answer to my obesity. Knowing this, I was still impatient, so I came up with a mantra: *This weight no longer belongs to me; I have released it. It will just take some time to shed it from my physical body.* A positive attitude and sticking to the plan 100 percent has really helped me tremendously, as has interacting with others trying to lose weight on my blog: **MeandJorge.com**.

When you hit a plateau, start the plan over again like it's Day 1. Reread your favorite sections of the book; if you kept a food log or diary, reread it, too. What were you doing then that you aren't doing now? Stop using any specialty products you've discovered or foods you've added back, and go back to the basics. I personally think that when a diet stops working for us, in actuality we have stopped working the diet.

On my blog, I am often asked if people can do this plan but keep using artificial sweeteners. I always answer that if you don't give up the artificial

Amber
Lost 54 pounds!

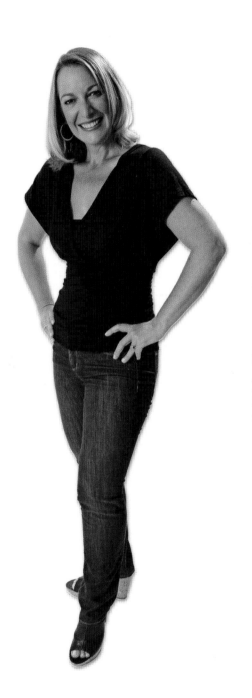

sweeteners, you will never lose the taste for sugar and the cravings it creates. It teaches your taste buds that everything you consume should be extremely sweet. Going cold turkey on artificial sweeteners is the only way to do it. I've seen dozens of readers on my blog try to taper off or have it occasionally, and it never works. For myself, the fear of giving up my diet sodas was much, much worse than actually just doing it.

What's Next?

The reward I feel from sharing my story and how it helps people feels just as good as losing all the weight. With my newfound energy and passion for writing, I'm going to continue to share my advice on my blog.

My Best Tip

Don't overthink the plan or you will become overwhelmed by how much weight you want to lose. Instead of thinking, *I can't do this forever,* ask yourself, *Can I eat this way for the rest of the day?* then *Can I do this again tomorrow?* Treat your cravings like the addiction they are, and just take it one meal and day at a time. Before you know it, you'll be at your goal weight.

FAST TRACK
SUCCESS
STORY

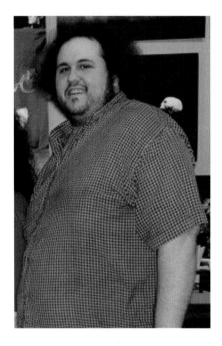

Before

Age: 25
Height: 6'0"
Pounds Lost: 210

I'm a 25-year-old from the Jersey Shore, living my dream of being a full-time professional musician and theater performer. As happy as I was to be onstage, I felt like my extra weight was holding me back from being the best performer possible. By April 1, 2009, I had reached my heaviest weight of 375 pounds. I knew it was time for a change.

My first attempt to lose the weight involved giving the South Beach Diet a try, but I wasn't impressed because I didn't like using all the artificial sweeteners. Even so, the low-sugar and low-carb idea was the only thing that made sense to me. I started to lose a little bit of weight on that diet, but it came in fits and starts . . . and at the end of the day, I still didn't really know what to eat or why.

Thankfully, I stumbled upon Jorge's Belly Fat Cure through Amber's (page 16) blog. I followed along with Amber on her journey to reach a healthy goal weight, finding great foods and converting to stevia in my coffee and cooking. *The Belly Fat Cure* made so much sense to me in a user-friendly, personal, and inviting way.

By taking it up a notch with the Fast Track program, I've now lost more than 200 pounds! I'm so much more confident that I even went out and joined a gym to work on toning, maintaining, and strengthening my body.

Ever since Jorge showed me how dangerous and fattening sugar is, and how it is hidden in so

Anthony
Lost 210 pounds!

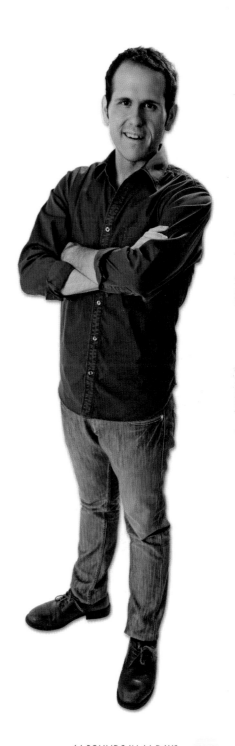

many of the foods we have always been told were healthy, my life has been completely different. Not only do I look and feel better, but I have more energy to pour into my passion in life: performing.

What's Next?

Now that I'm at a healthy weight, I'm looking to perform even more and in a wider variety of roles. I also feel for the first time in my life that I have the health and energy I need to travel and experience the world more. Traveling has always been a dream of mine, but it seemed out of reach, given those 200-plus pounds of extra baggage . . . but not anymore!

My Best Tip

Not that long ago, losing 200 pounds seemed impossible to me. By pushing that disbelief aside and focusing on what I *could* accomplish instead of what I couldn't, the impossible came true. So no matter how much or how little weight *you* want to lose, you absolutely can do it with this program if you just believe in yourself!

FAST TRACK
SUCCESS STORY

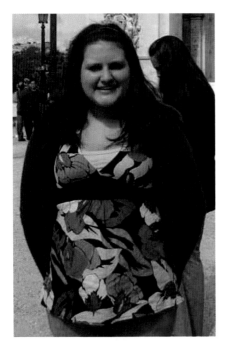

Before

Age: 18
Height: 5'3"
Pounds Lost: 66

I was the youngest of three girls in a family where meals were typically fast food, and nutrition was not a priority. Then a few years ago, I was diagnosed with fatty liver disease and tried to lose weight with Optifast. My mom, older sister, and I were all trying to lose weight together, but it turned out to be just a temporary fix. It wasn't long before I had gained back even more weight than I had lost.

When my mom first heard about *The Belly Fat Cure,* she downloaded a free menu and information packet from Jorge's website . . . but then she forgot about it. Luckily, I found the printouts one day and started following the program on my own. My family immediately noticed the changes in both my appearance and choices, and they were all amazed! I had suddenly gone from the girl who used to hide in baggy clothes to the girl who loved to get dressed up and express herself.

One by one, my example motivated my family members to believe that they could do it, too, and now we are fully committed to making this a lifestyle change we are doing together. Today, we are all completely different and so much happier. Not just kind of happier—I mean a million times happier! To know that I had something to do with that, even though I'm just the baby of the family, gives me a feeling I can't even describe. Jorge

Jessica
Lost 66 pounds!

changed my life, and then he and I changed my family's life. Thank you so much!

What's Next?

College is right around the corner for me, and it may seem kind of silly, but I can't wait to break the myth of the freshman 15! In fact, I plan on losing another 15 pounds my freshman year. I've also had such a great experience getting my family involved with healthier eating that I'm working on spreading the message to all my friends . . . it helps that they're all begging to learn my secrets!

My Best Tip

Being 17 when I started the program, I thought veggies were unappealing—but Jorge showed me how to dress them up into rich and tasty Super Carbs with butter and other delicious flavors. It wasn't long before I actually started to experience cravings for foods such as broccoli! When you use butter to make healthy foods more exciting, pretty soon your cravings shift toward those guilt-free foods.

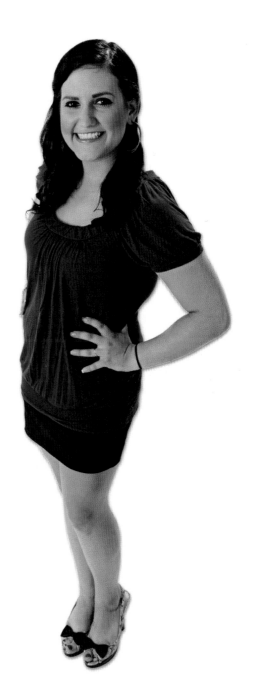

FAST TRACK
SUCCESS
STORY

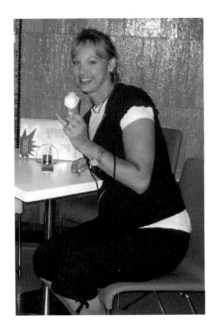

Before

Age: 40
Height: 5'8"
Pounds Lost: 27

Like most moms, my kids took priority over my belly fat. I was really athletic when I was younger, and even though I gained some weight while taking care of my family, I didn't think much of it. Because I always thought it took a lot of time and energy to stay fit, and I had responsibilities as a mother, I was sure I would never have the time to lose weight again.

Even more depressing was the notion that once we women reach 40, those "last 20 pounds" become impossible to lose. I feel as if most women just accept that extra weight after a certain age, and I thought I would end up doing the same. I worried that if I did accept those 20 pounds, I would accept 10 more . . . and then another 10. . . .

Luckily, the Fast Track taught me that it's not about making sacrifices with your time and energy, but only about making *smart* choices. These smart choices Jorge taught me totally fit the lifestyle I already had, and were key to getting back into the body I feel most comfortable in. Also, with the extra energy I've discovered since losing the weight, I actually have *more* quality time to devote to my family. What started out as an attempt to feel a little better in my clothes has actually improved my ability to be the best mom I can be. Bonus!

Alicia
Lost 27 pounds!

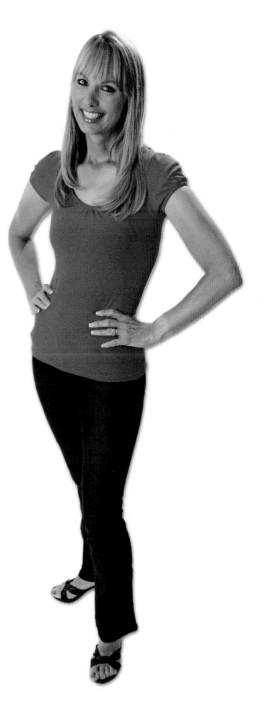

What's Next?

As a mother with teenage daughters, my goal is to be the best role model possible. Young girls have so much pressure put on them to look a certain way, but I want my girls to know that it is their faith and their health that really matter. This program has helped me learn how to be healthier, and it makes me proud that I can now share this with my kids.

My Best Tip

Be patient, especially right at the beginning. If you follow the program, it won't take long to get the first payoff that will empower you and give you the momentum to make it all the way to your goal weight. Let every pound you lose be the motivation to lose the next one!

FAST TRACK
SUCCESS
STORY

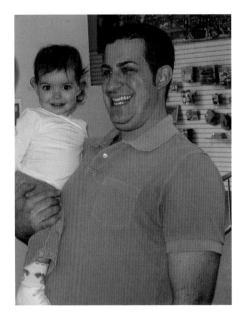

Before

Age: 34
Height: 5'10"
Pounds Lost: 33

In January 2010, I weighed in at 208 pounds. Despite a relentless routine of exercising six days each week, my weight had ballooned out of control. I had no handle on my nutrition at all. As I was exercising so much, I was basically eating whatever and whenever I wanted. I actually thought I was eating healthy by eating lots of low-fat and fat-free foods. I needed to take control of my nutrition.

I heard about *The Belly Fat Cure* through a helpful friend, and as soon as I read it, the science made perfect sense to me. I realized the foods I was eating were *loaded* with hidden sugars, and that was making me fatter and fatter.

I started on the program and the weight began melting away. I think I lost 10 or 12 pounds in just the first week! I continued my exercise program as usual, and within the last five months, I have lost 33 pounds. I am now leaner and fitter than I have ever been. I have never been stronger or felt better, and lost five inches off my waist!

Dr. Wilensky
Lost 33 pounds!

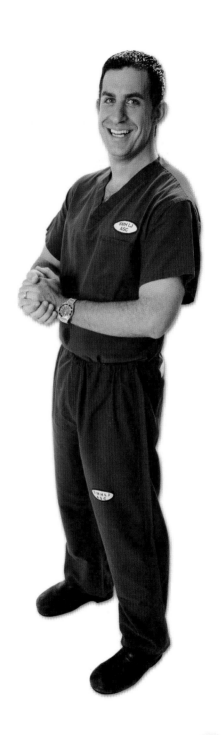

What's Next?

With my newfound energy, I have taken my physical activity to entirely new levels. A group of friends and I will be hiking the Grand Canyon in a 47-mile, rim-to-rim-to-rim hike this fall, and I can't wait!

My Best Tip

A lot of us, especially guys, think we can eat whatever we want so long as we exercise like fiends. From my personal experience and education, I know for a fact that this is a myth. It is all about what you eat, not how hard you work it off, that determines your true health and weight. Once you figure that out and eat the right foods, exercise changes from a chore to something fun.

FAST TRACK
SUCCESS
STORY

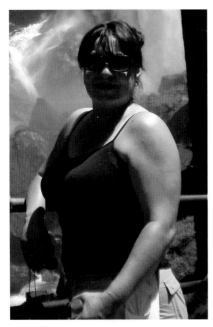

Before

Age: 50
Height: 5'3"
Pounds Lost: 15

Doing the Fast Track has truly been a life-changing experience! I have a family history of high cholesterol, high blood pressure, and diabetes. I had been taking medication for my high LDL (also called the "bad cholesterol") levels and triglycerides for more than 20 years, but had little success in maintaining them at normal levels even while on medication. My doctors had been telling me that my body just naturally overproduces bad cholesterol and triglycerides, and that I would have to take medication for the rest of my life as a result. I have always eaten pretty healthfully and have maintained an exercise regimen of three to four times per week at the gym as part of my lifestyle, but my cholesterol values still remained high.

The opportunity came to try Jorge's Fast Track edition of the Belly Fat Cure in San Diego, so I decided I would see what it was all about. At the first meeting, our group was given a list of foods we would be allowed to eat: whole eggs, bacon, sausage, butter, vegetables, and meats. Well, my first reaction was, "Oh no! I can't eat eggs, bacon, or sausage, let alone butter." I was certain my triglyceride values, which were already at an insane 428, would shoot up even more after eating these foods. But after listening to Jorge talk about foods that are packed with hidden sugars,

Haydee
Lowered triglycerides by 258!

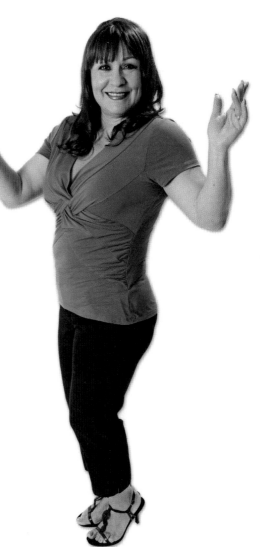

and about lowering insulin levels in order to achieve weight loss, I decided to go forward with the challenge.

I had my blood work checked before the final meeting, and to my surprise, my triglycerides had gone from 428 . . . to 170! I was ecstatic! These were the lowest numbers I'd ever had, and I did it without medication. In a sense, I actually lowered my triglycerides by trading statins for butter! It sounds crazy, but it's true!

What's Next?

So many of my family members are taking statins that it is my goal to help each and every one of them use food as medicine to correct the problem.

My Best Tip

You must learn to question all your assumptions if you want to be successful, since so much of what you have been told is wrong!

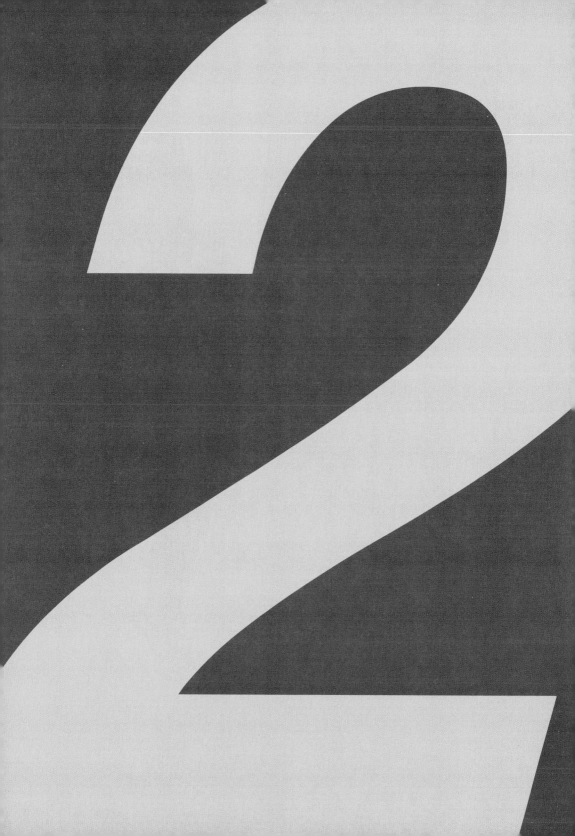

The Ultimate
Carb Swap

"Carbohydrate controls insulin; insulin controls fat storage."

— **MARK SISSON,** author of *The Primal Blueprint*

You know what hidden sugar does to your body: it grows belly fat. Sugar grows belly fat, ages you inside and out, and lays the foundation for three of the biggest killers in our modern era: heart disease, cancer, and diabetes. That single fact is the central, revolutionary truth at the heart of *The Belly Fat Cure.* The difference with this Fast Track edition lies in how closely we look for insulin-stimulating sugar in *all* its forms.

It takes little imagination to understand that **simple carbohydrates** (street name: sugar) and **complex carbohydrates** (street name: carbs) are really slightly different versions of the

Simple carbohydrates:
Most commonly referred to as sugar and quickly absorbed into the bloodstream, simple carbohydrates drive the production of insulin and feed the blood-sugar roller coaster.

Complex carbohydrates:
Although these are absorbed more slowly, even complex carbs will eventually become simple carbs and drive the production of insulin. All carbs will cut in line as a fuel source, ensuring that the body never taps into stored fat . . . exactly why weight loss is accelerated when carbs come from only the most ideal sources.

same thing. If you read your food labels, you will notice that sugar is counted twice: first as sugar and then again as carbohydrates, because sugar is a form of carbohydrate. Even though complex carbohydrates impact insulin to a lesser degree, they always impact insulin! No matter how healthy they may look, all carbohydrates are broken down by your body into their simple, sugary form.

So in order to accelerate your results, you will need to use the Ultimate Carb Swap to ensure that *all* the carbs you eat are of the highest value. But how can you get rid of more of the sneaky insulin-stimulating carbohydrates that are hiding in your meals? With a little more digging into human biology and history, the answer becomes abundantly clear:

To accelerate your weight loss from 4 to 7 pounds a week, you must simply *remove grains and starch* from your lifestyle for 14 days.

Now don't put this book down just yet! Even my most loyal clients have had quite a reaction to the previous statement, so I'm sure that you are thinking one (or all) of the following:

- *But whole grains are vital for good health! They protect my heart . . . haven't you seen those Cheerios commercials?*

- *But grains are the foundation of the food pyramid!*

- *I love bread and pasta so much; I can't trade them in to lose weight!*

- *I'll get constipated if I don't eat grains!*

- *My goodness, is this just Atkins all over again? I already tried that and gained it all back!*

All of these concerns and more will be addressed throughout this chapter, but you must first open your mind to the possibility that the cornerstone of what we have been told is a "balanced diet" may not be helping you lose weight. If you continue to read the facts I present throughout this chapter with an open mind, you can unlock the true nature of your relationship with starches and give your body the boost it needs to release weight at a potentially accelerated rate.

It's important that I point something out here: although I believe that the Fast Track program works quite well as an ongoing lifestyle that delivers amazing weight loss and health results, it may not be a perfect fit for absolutely *everyone.* Many clients use this program as a way to kick-start weight loss, break through a plateau, or simply as additional knowledge they use to get the most from the Belly Fat Cure. Before you decide how it may fit into your life, all I ask is that you try following the Fast Track program faithfully for only 14 days.

> ***Opioids:***
> *Any external substance that numbs pain and creates a feeling of euphoria, typically by mimicking the body's endorphins and often leading to dependence.*

In order to accelerate, you must first believe that you can survive without grains and starches for 14 days. And you will—you won't just survive, but thrive! The reason your "instinct" tells you that this is impossible results from the fact that sugar, starches, and grains resemble drug-like **opioids,** meaning that they mimic your body's own **endorphins,** binding to brain receptors that make you feel happy. This is similar to how the drugs heroin and opium cause humans to feel better . . . at least temporarily.

> ***Endorphins:***
> *The body's mechanism for feeling blissful, this compound binds to receptor sites in the brain and induces a natural sense of well-being.*

My favorite study demonstrating the pain-numbing effects of sugar involved rats given varying amounts of sugar to keep their paws on a hot plate. The rats given the most sugar kept their paws on the hot plate the longest, because they felt the least pain. A recently published review in *Neuroscience & Biobehavioral Reviews* found that sugar and drugs cause similar changes in the limbic system of the brain! Rats that had sugar included in their diet and were then forced to abstain from sugar even exhibited opiate-like withdrawal symptoms.

So if you are having a negative reaction to the idea of cutting grains and starches out of your meals because you "love" them too darn much, consider that an indicator of how your body has grown accustomed to the comforting feeling these convenient foods deliver every few hours. There are varying degrees of carb cravings, and I address strategies for overcoming both the physical and psychological aspects of these cravings in Chapter 7.

Super Carbs:
Low-sugar vegetables that provide you with the ideal source of carbohydrates and dietary fiber while also providing balance to your body's pH.

Don't feel guilty if you have used sugar or grains as a way to feel better, because you're not alone. Anytime I've ever asked a group of successful clients if they can relate to such a scenario, about 98 percent of the people in the room have raised their hands. The good news is that most were able to break free of their addictions while learning the meal-preparation secrets to make the good **Super Carbs** taste just as yummy, and in only a few minutes . . . and you can, too!

Health: Your History, Your Destiny

The most crucial argument against the belief that sugar, grains, and starches (especially when they're in the form of processed products) form the basis of an ideal diet comes not just from the latest cutting-edge research, but from a look into our distant past.

There are many biologists who understand health to be something that an organism creates **when its environment most closely resembles the circumstances for**

which its genes were selected. That's a fancy way of saying that whatever "niche" an organism was designed to fill is the one where that organism will experience the greatest happiness and well-being. Humans are just another kind of organism, so it would hold true that our own genetics produce abundant health when our environment (including our diet and lifestyle) most closely resembles the hunter-gatherer lifestyle from which we all originated.

This is the core philosophy behind a style of eating often referred to as either the Caveman or **Paleolithic diet,** and I am not the first to float the idea that the answers to what we should eat reside quite clearly in our origins. If you were to say that the recommendations in the Fast Track program are very similar to Atkins, I'd say

> ***Paleolithic diet:***
> *A diet based on the nutrition available to the human species more than 10,000 years ago. This diet restricts foods that only became available due to modern agricultural and industrial processes.*

you were considerably off, and I'll reveal more differences later in the book. If you drew on the similarities between the Fast Track program and a Paleolithic approach, however, you would be closer to the truth.

I strongly believe that nourishing our bodies with the mix of foods our genes were selected for is this century's answer to the question of "What do I eat?" **But I also know that no one wants to live like a caveman in these modern times.** We couldn't live like Paleolithic humans even if we wanted: we are like perfectly engineered aircraft that find ourselves drifting in the open ocean, unable to return to the sky. Our only option is to adapt to our surroundings as best we can, a skill at which humanity is actually quite adept. That is the challenge of this approach: navigating this marvelously modern world and making choices that are both in line with our dietary history and incredibly satisfying and easy. So no, eating like our ancestors doesn't mean eating bugs or passing on cheese—it just means having vegetables and meat make up the bulk of our diet.

Many of my clients weren't surprised to discover that temporarily removing grains and starches from their diets would help them lose weight, but they expressed the belief that it was somehow unhealthy. "It's not balanced," some told me. "I'll cut out bread and pasta for a day or two, but anything more than that isn't safe." **This idea that a meal remains unbalanced without a grain or starch is one that I would like to change.** When we gain an accurate perspective of the history of grains as part of our diet, the belief that we must eat them at every meal begins to change. Although agriculture brought limited grains to humanity around 10,000 years ago, it seems as though it's a friendship that has stood the test of time. Zoom out some, though, and the picture changes: grains have been a part of our lifestyle for less than one percent of our time on Earth.

That means that for thousands of generations, essentially the entirety of our history, humans and their ancestors flourished while eating minimal to no grains. Using the biological view of health I mentioned earlier, it becomes clear that having grains and starches at every turn is not in alignment with our DNA. There simply wasn't enough time for humans to have adapted to the changes in diet and environment that have taken place in just the last 10,000 years.

When you take into account that we have been eating processed sugar and *processed* grains in the amounts we do today for only about 200 years (since the Industrial Revolution), it's clear that today's average diet is one that our bodies have been subjected to for only .01 percent of our time on Earth. This shock to our systems is at the root of nearly all modern diseases that plague industrialized nations.

Evidence supporting a healthy lifestyle free of sugar and grains doesn't stop at the fact that humanity survived without them for more than 99 percent of our history. Anthropologists who study our ancestors have noticed a change in the fossil record before and after the shift from hunting and gathering to farming: at the same time that a society experienced a proliferation in agriculture and began relying more heavily on grains, its citizens could expect a decrease in average life span, decreased stature, an increase in bone mineral disorders, and even a decrease in average brain size. Some scientists believe that the change in diet could have been the cause of all these effects, resulting from grains displacing the plants and vegetables these societies had previously been foraging.

Grains and Osteoporosis

Although grains do contain calcium, you can experience bone loss and osteoporosis if you rely too heavily on them in your diet. This happens as a result of a phenomenon that is all too often overlooked: **calcium balance.**

Calcium balance:
Not just how much calcium you consume, but how much you absorb and how much you retain. Healthy calcium balance is aided by vitamin D, magnesium, and alkalizing foods.

Most women I talk to have never heard of calcium balance, even though it is much more important for bone strength than calcium intake. Calcium balance determines your body's ability to hold on to the bones you have, and is dictated by the balance of acidic and **alkalizing** foods in the diet.

Throughout humanity's history, we didn't need to worry about alkalinity and acidity— even though we ate an abundance of animal products (which are acidic), we naturally balanced the acidity by consuming an equal amount of alkaline plants and vegetables. The problem began when we started consuming too much sugar and grain, which are also acidic. Replacing more and more alkaline plants with acidic grains in our diet has led to higher and higher levels of

Alkalizing:
Foods that bring balance to your body's pH by causing your system to become more alkaline after digestion. Plants like Super Carbs are your body's ideal alkalizing foods.

acidity in the body. In order to balance pH, the body has needed to tap into some other source of alkalinity: calcium from bones.

When you consume a diet that is too acidic, one way your body will try to balance it is by eating at the bones in order to get at the alkaline calcium they are made of. For this reason, **swapping acidic grains for alkaline Super Carbs is one of the most important steps women can take to maintain bone health and defeat osteoporosis.**

Other Negative Contributors

Celiac disease offers a glimpse into the most extreme example of what happens when our bodies reject foods they weren't intended to eat. Whether you have celiac disease or not, it could be very helpful to at least consider that your body may not have completely adapted to the changes in the human diet of the last 200 or even 10,000 years.

You've probably heard of the gluten-free diet, which is prescribed to treat those with full-blown celiac disease. It is estimated that about one percent, or three million Americans, have celiac disease. Yet of those three million people, a shocking 97 percent of them are undiagnosed.

People with celiac disease cannot tolerate even small amounts of **gluten,** which is a protein found in wheat, rye, and barley, and even in some makeup and medicines. The symptoms of celiac disease vary from person to person, with some people showing no outward symptoms at all. Lack of symptoms, however, does not mean a lack of harm. When people with celiac disease eat anything containing gluten, their digestive system attacks itself. The resulting damage makes it very difficult for the body to absorb nutrients, leading to nutritional deficiencies that can cause a whole host of dreadful diseases. Many people experience what is known as "gluten sensitivity," so even those without full-blown celiac disease may find that gluten has caused silent damage to their digestive system.

A similar protein you may not have heard about is called **lectin,** which is found in grains and legumes (beans), and can adversely affect some people much like gluten. Some researchers believe that lectin may interact with cells in the body and potentially interfere with metabolism and hormone balance in certain individuals. Still other scientists believe lectin may also interfere with processes of the immune system in some people, instigating attacks that have been linked to **autoimmune disorders.** The American Autoimmune Related Diseases Association reports that approximately 50 million Americans suffer from autoimmune disorders,

> *Lectin:*
> *A protein found in foods like grains and legumes (beans) that recent studies have suggested may cause damage to the digestive system and resistance to the hormone leptin, which is a key hormone that regulates metabolism. Leptin resistance may lead to obesity in some.*

> *Autoimmune disorders:*
> *Disorders that arise from the immune system attacking normal cells in the body. Common autoimmune disorders include arthritis, psoriasis, narcolepsy, lupus, multiple sclerosis, and perhaps even schizophrenia and Alzheimer's. Many now believe the underlying cause of these diseases is incorrect diet.*

including Hashimoto's thyroiditis, lupus, multiple sclerosis, and type 1 diabetes. (Fibromyalgia and Parkinson's disease are also suspected by some to be autoimmune disorders, but this has yet to be confirmed.)

I certainly don't share any of this information because I wish to scare you. For so many people, choosing healthy whole grains and legumes can be a fantastically successful strategy . . . that's why I created the Belly Fat Cure! However, other people may also benefit tremendously from uncovering an unknown reaction to the foods we eliminate in the Fast Track program. No matter which category you fall into at the end of your 14-day challenge, you will have gained a deeper wisdom of how the food you put into your mouth interacts with your unique body.

Release Misinformation, Release Belly Fat

If fat truly is our ideal source of fuel, why do we associate energy with grains and starches like pasta, bread, and potatoes? There are two major reasons that explain why our society places such a disproportionate emphasis on these foods instead of vegetables and meat. The first is the fact that we only recently even visited the idea that these foods might not be the most healthful for some people. To be fair, 10,000 years does seem like an awfully long time to most of us, but in this case perspective is everything.

The second reason has more to do with the information we've been served up by Conventional Wisdom, Inc., for 60 years. While I will refrain from theorizing that there is a conspiracy by big business to keep us hooked on only the most profitable foods, I will point out that food products made from grains are better for business in a number of ways. Their shelf life is much longer than other foods like meat, veggies, and eggs, which means that food conglomerates lose less money on products going bad.

Add to that the fact that our tax dollars are used to heavily subsidize grains in the form of the **Farm Bill,** and suddenly corn and wheat products simply become the smartest, most economical choice for food. However, it is all an illusion. The corn and wheat industries sell their products cheaply because they receive billions of our tax dollars to keep prices low, a situation that has helped finance the increase in the prevalence of high-fructose corn syrup in the American diet by 1,000 percent since 1970.

So, for just two weeks, I'd like you to just explore the idea that grains and starches *may not* form the healthy foundation of *your* balanced diet as you've been told countless times. Will you consider that your health and body can improve dramatically by creating a

> **Farm Bill:**
> *The primary agricultural and food-policy tool of the federal government, in which billions of dollars are given to farmers as subsidies. The majority of the subsidies go toward some of the least ideal foods: corn, wheat, soybeans, and rice.*

modern lifestyle that more closely resembles that of your ancestors? If you can answer "Yes," then you are *almost* ready to lose as close to 14 pounds in 14 days as is possible for your body.

By swapping your old standbys of sugar, starches, and grains for the Super Carbs found in the best green veggies, you will jump-start a metabolism that has lain dormant your entire life. Releasing the myth that grains are absolutely required for health is the final piece of the puzzle when it comes to boosting your levels of fat-melting **glucagon** to their peak, and the key to accelerating your weight loss.

The temporary absence of grains from your lifestyle could create one more hurdle to overcome, but also an opportunity for the Fast Track program to correct one of the many shortcomings of all those "low carb" diets that

> **Glucagon:**
> *The body's mechanism for shrinking fat tissue, this hormone is only capable of unlocking energy from fat cells when insulin is low.*

came before. **What about fiber?** The next chapter tackles the final weight-loss myth standing in your way to success, and will give you the last breakthrough you need to ensure a smooth transition to your new metabolism and body.

FAST TRACK
SUCCESS
STORY

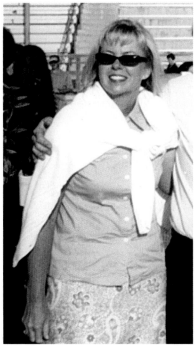

Before

Age: 46
Height: 5'3"
Pounds Lost: 25

I have struggled with my weight ever since I was a child. From ages 6 to 12 I was a "chubby" kid, until a friend and I decided to lose some weight because, well, we had discovered boys. With great effort I managed to stay pretty thin until I turned 40, when my weight started to creep up. By 50, I had put on an extra 25 pounds.

In addition to this, I'd feel bloated and have to unfasten my pants by evening every day. Since my mother had this same issue and I'd read that women over 40 often experience this weight gain and bloating, I felt resigned to this uncomfortable way of life.

During the last few years, I've tried Weight Watchers, Nutrisystem, and Atkins. Yet whenever I tried those diets, I'd get horrible headaches during the first few days and either try to live through it or quit. I always felt like I was starving and couldn't sleep. Nutrisystem was the worst for me because it drastically increased the horrible gas and bloating I was already suffering from!

When I had a hysterectomy last fall, I put on even more weight. When I expressed an interest in losing the excess pounds, a friend told me that this is just how it is once you have a hysterectomy. So many women my age resign themselves to being overweight, and I did not want to be a part of that!

In a stroke of luck, I bought a *First for Women* magazine at the grocery store. It compared a few diets, and the Belly Fat Cure sounded reasonable and like something that I could do. I looked at

Darla
Lost 25 pounds!

Jorge's site online as well, bought his book, and connected with him on Facebook, which is where I heard about the Fast Track program. Within a few days of starting the program, I noticed that the gas and bloating were completely gone. I lost two inches off of my waist within the first week and had no headaches! In fact, I have not had one headache since being on the Fast Track, which is unheard of for me. On top of that, the waistline I had ten years ago is back, and I'm thrilled.

What's Next?

One by one, I'm determined to motivate all my girlfriends to change their attitudes and start the Belly Fat Cure.

My Best Tip

If you're over 40, you're not stuck being overweight. But if you resign yourself to being overweight, you will always be overweight. All you have to do is believe in yourself and follow Jorge's recommendations, and everything else will fall back into place!

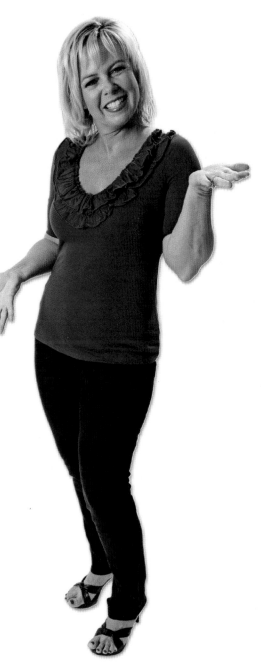

FAST TRACK
SUCCESS STORY

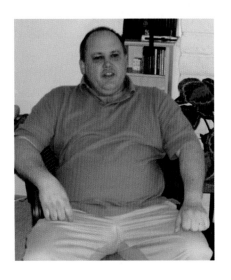

Before

Age: 48
Height: 5'7"
Pounds Lost: 32

Before starting the Belly Fat Cure, it was hard to get out of bed without excruciating aches and pains from being overweight, having a blood clot in my leg, and overall poor eating habits. Every night someone in my family would bring home two or three bags of fast food, and we'd all sit around the television eating junk that was slowly poisoning us.

Now I have more energy to perform on the job and can even work on projects at home without being physically or mentally drained. I also enjoy preparing and eating food much more because I can actually feel how this style of eating improves my mood, energy, and memory. I have lost all desire for the sugar-packed foods that were the mainstay of my diet for 48 years. My family and I owe our health and renewed energy to Jorge Cruise, the Belly Fat Cure, and his amazingly supportive team of coaches!

What's Next?

My immediate family is now 142 pounds lighter thanks to the Belly Fat Cure and the Fast Track program, and we are all still losing. Now we want to share the secret with the rest of our family and see just how much healthier and happier we can all be. I'm also

Chris
Lost 32 pounds!

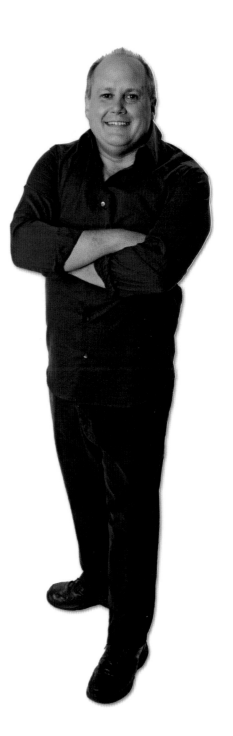

looking forward to getting outdoors and being active more often. I went on a hike with my fellow Fast Tracker and new buddy Karl (page 200) recently, which he told me would be two miles. Afterward, he admitted that we'd actually walked about seven miles . . . I couldn't believe that I was enjoying myself so much that I didn't even notice!

My Best Tip

Keep it simple and ready to go! Our family fridge is stocked with precooked chicken-breast strips and pre-prepped veggies so that making meals takes five minutes max. Not having enough time to eat well was my biggest excuse, and now it's gone!

FAST TRACK
SUCCESS
STORY

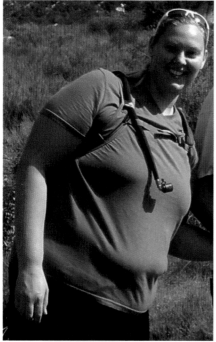

Before

Age: 28
Height: 6'3"
Pounds Lost: 61

Before the Fast Track, I thought I was on my way to being another story in my family's history of diabetes and heart disease . . . not really exciting thoughts for a 28-year-old to have. I had hit 345 pounds, and my doctor prescribed a low-fat diet to reduce my cholesterol concerns and more exercise to lose weight, but the number on the scale stayed the same.

Then last year I got a call from my sister, who told me to run to Costco and pick up a copy of *The Belly Fat Cure.* I was shocked to discover the real source of my problem: hidden sugar! How was I supposed to know how much sugar was in milk? It turns out that it *doesn't* do a body good!

Now I feel completely empowered! I have realized that we can inherit unhealthy habits from our families, but not genes that condemn us to being sick and overweight . . . that is just an excuse! All the discoveries Jorge shared with me, and especially the easy-to-understand way he framed them, have made me feel in charge of my health for the first time in my life. After believing for so long that losing weight was a near-impossible battle that required tremendous sacrifice and hard work, I feel liberated to know the truth: it is actually really easy!

Christy
Lost 61 pounds!

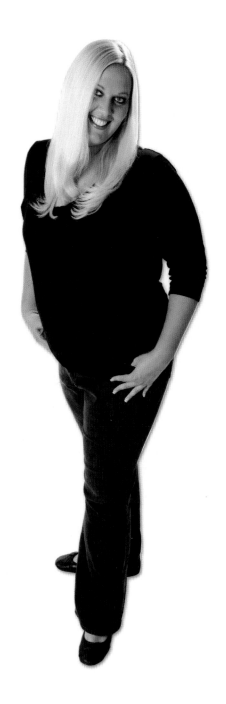

What's Next?

I still have quite a bit of weight to lose before I reach my goal, but I've continued to lose weight each week ever since I experienced the most dramatic results during those first two weeks. I've decided to stick to the Fast Track program, but not just until I reach my goal—it will be for the rest of my life. Understanding how this way of eating isn't just a way to lose weight but can also lead to better health and energy makes being motivated to stick with it so easy.

My Best Tip

Follow the plan exactly as it is written! I told myself I wasn't going to ask questions or try to change the plan, and my results were amazing. In fact, sticking to the plan exactly made it even easier. I also recommend finding an outlet for all the extra energy that will be coming your way once you make it through the 14-day challenge. I had so much energy that I started working out, and I really believe that this has kept my results to the maximum!

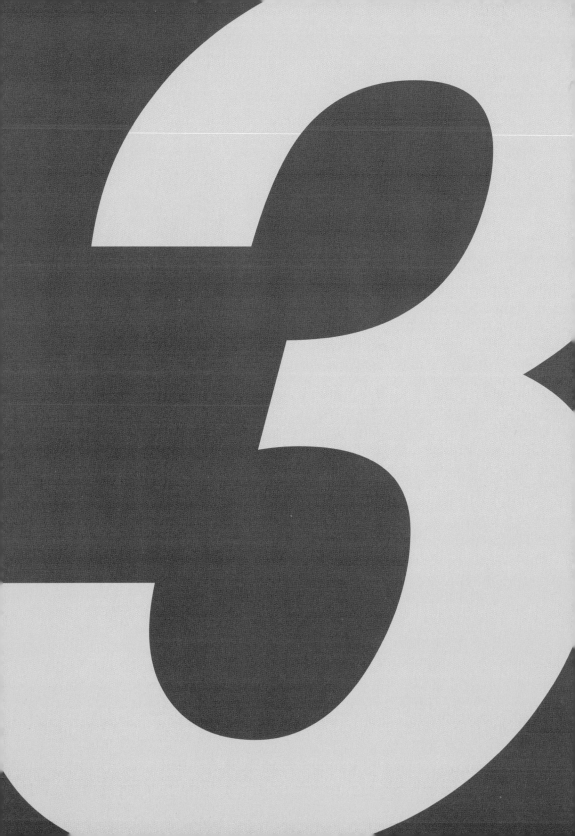

3 Ensuring Your Success

"The flora has a collective metabolic activity equal to a virtual organ within an organ . . ."

— **ANN O'HARA AND FERGUS SHANAHAN,**
University College Cork, National University of Ireland

This chapter may prove to be the most surprising yet, because I'm going to address head-on the trendiest superstar of weight loss there is today. While there is a growing chorus of experts who are sounding the alarm that insulin is the key to practically everything, you may be hard-pressed to find someone else in the mainstream tackling the final misunderstanding that

> *The fiber myth:*
> *The belief that essential dietary fiber and "high-fiber food products" made from grains are the same thing.*

can prevent you from reinventing yourself: **the fiber myth.**

Dietary fiber is an absolutely critical element to your health, diet, and weight loss. In fact, it is really the most popular and accepted weight-loss message of the last decade—and you will hear me continue to echo that message. However, a problem arises when food companies and marketing campaigns take advantage of our desire for more fiber to encourage us to buy their unhealthy products.

My favorite example is when Kellogg claimed that the fiber in Frosted Mini-Wheats increased children's attentiveness by 20 percent. The Federal Trade Commission ordered the untruthful marketing claims to be discontinued, but I can imagine that many parents leapt at the opportunity to increase the fiber in their family's diet. In this example, Kellogg tried to sell consumers on the fiber but stuck them with a bill of 12 sugar grams, 3 carb servings, and high-fructose corn syrup. It should come as no surprise that this recipe failed to foster attentive children.

With the Fast Track program, I challenge you to question the conventional wisdom of health and weight loss, just like I asked you to do in *The Belly Fat Cure*. Remember when you first realized that fat-free peach yogurt was actually fattening? Here is the next step of your awakening:

**The *source* of fiber is just as important
as the *amount* of fiber.**

Sound familiar? Just like calories, all fiber grams are not created equal. The Ultimate Carb Swap is such a powerful tool for accelerated weight loss because it focuses your attention on fiber from the most ideal and nutrient-dense sources: Super Carbs! In the Belly Best Food List in Chapter 6, I've identified those Super Carbs that are especially rich in fiber and extremely effective at clearing false belly fat and promoting regularity.

So we all love fiber, especially when it comes from vegetables like broccoli. That's the end of the story, right? Not quite. What if fiber is great at addressing the *symptoms* of digestive problems, but fails to correct the actual *cause* of the irregularity in many people? Hopefully, by now you have become more comfortable with exchanging stale assumptions from the past for new perspectives on weight loss. In this chapter, **you will learn how to treat the cause of your digestive issues, rather than just the symptoms.** This key ingredient truly makes the Fast Track program a unique and ultimate evolution of what many people refer to dismissively as the "**low-carb diet.**"

> **Dysbacteriosis:**
> A condition widely overlooked in the West in which the gut loses its bacterial microflora, becoming sterile and unable to function as intended. Common disorders that result from dysbacteriosis include constipation and suppressed immune function. A deficiency in vitamin K, which is secreted by healthy flora, has also been linked to osteoporosis and coronary heart disease.

Dysbacteriosis: The Overlooked Epidemic

Dysbacteriosis describes a very common condition in which the beneficial **gut flora** that live inside our digestive system have been severely damaged or completely obliterated. We then tend to turn to fiber supplements and eat high-fiber foods in an attempt to regain digestive regularity. However,

> **Gut flora:**
> The collection of microorganisms living in the human gut with which our bodies have evolved a symbiotic relationship. It is estimated that there are about 500 species living in the human body, and they perform metabolic activities that many compare to that of an organ.

there wouldn't be so much pressure to add ever-increasing amounts of roughage to our diets if we recognized the important role that intestinal bacteria plays in digestion. Allow me to introduce you to a few billion new friends who would like nothing more than to help you better digest food and lose weight.

Symbiotic:
A relationship between two organisms in which one or both benefit from the functions of the other.

Our bodies have developed over thousands of generations to rely on the **symbiotic** relationship between our intestines and the microflora that live inside it. The surface area of the human intestinal tract is about equal to that of a tennis court, and is covered by a thin film of this helpful, good bacteria. In healthy individuals, intestinal bacteria can account for three to five pounds of body weight! This flora is so incredibly vital to optimal health and performs so many functions in our body that many doctors speak of it as an "organ," in the same way that blood and skin are organs.

**In this light, dysbacteriosis means that your body
is missing a five-pound vital organ—and without it,
it cannot effectively digest food and eliminate waste.**

We turn to **supplemental fiber** in an attempt to replace one of the most important (but not only) functions of our missing gut flora: retaining water in stools.

Supplemental fiber:
Soluble or insoluble fiber that is added to the diet as a means of promoting healthy digestion. While also part of a healthy lifestyle, this may not correct the underlying cause of irregularity or poor digestion.

Fiber absorbs water and grows to five times its size and weight, mimicking the role normally reserved for the bacteria in a healthy gut. So while fiber assists in healthy digestion, it cannot completely replace healthy flora. Also, potential consequences may arise from using too much fiber as a means of moving the bowels. Once again, we must understand that there can always be too much of a good thing:

- **Intestinal inflammation.** The *excessive* presence of a substance your body is incapable of digesting may cause mechanical and chemical damage to the delicate lining of the intestines, leading to inflammation that inhibits the absorption of nutrients and can lead to acute deficiencies.

- **Intestinal disorders.** The inflammation mentioned above, which can result when excessive fiber provides the only means of moving the bowels, may lay the groundwork for irritable bowel syndrome (IBS) and the more serious inflammatory bowel disease (IBD). About 15 percent of Americans suffer from IBS, and two-thirds of them are women.

- **Leaky gut.** One of the most bizarre consequences of incorrect sources and amounts of fiber can be a condition called leaky gut. In this scenario, the "roughage" of too many indigestible food particles contributes to the damage and inflammation of the delicate intestinal lining I mentioned earlier. Once responsible for acting as a gatekeeper, the delicate lining is essentially sandpapered by excessive roughage and left with tiny "leaks." Rather than allowing only nutrients to pass through this thin barrier into your blood, larger particles, toxins, and bacteria can leak directly from the intestines into your bloodstream. Your body may confuse these particles for foreign invaders, setting off a body-wide inflammatory response that can worsen symptoms of IBS and may even contribute to autoimmune disorders like rheumatoid arthritis.

These conditions are indeed rare, and I still recommend a diet rich in the right kinds of fiber. However, I believe it is critical to illustrate what "too much of a good thing" might look like in the case of fiber. It also gives us a reason to seek the solution to the cause of conditions such as constipation, rather than to merely treat the symptoms with ever-increasing amounts of fiber.

Fixing the Problem vs. Covering It Up

The solution is simple: **treat the cause of the problem (dysbacteriosis) rather than covering up the symptoms (constipation) with more fiber from the wrong source.** But how do you know if you suffer from dysbacteriosis?

The most glaring red flag is an inability to move your bowels without the help of high-fiber grain products and supplements . . . which describes about 90 percent of my clients at the beginning of their 14-day challenge.

In order to ensure your fantastic success using the Ultimate Carb Swap—and because there are so many aspects of modern life that contribute to dysbacteriosis—I strongly advise that you assume a considerable amount of damage has already been done to your own gut flora. The good news is that, unlike most traditional organs in your body, you can actually regrow what has been lost. If you remain patient during the process of regrowing this lost organ and implement the following strategies to prevent dysbacteriosis and promote restoration, you will experience the most phenomenal results possible during your two-week transformation and beyond.

To avoid dysbacteriosis, you must first identify the aspects of modern life that kill off these vital friends of ours:

- **Antibiotics in meat and dairy.** Since modern agricultural practices often lead to overcrowded and sick animals, large doses of antibiotics are necessary to keep farm animals alive until slaughter. Traces of antibiotics make it into our food and thus into our bodies, damaging our beneficial gut flora. This is why I recommend that you choose hormone- and antibiotic-free animal products whenever you can.

- **Antibiotic medications.** While antibiotics can certainly save lives, they are often overprescribed. Even more problematic is that once the antibiotics are no longer necessary, the patient rarely takes the appropriate steps to restore the good bacteria that were destroyed along with the bad. One prescription of a powerful antibiotic can kill your entire population of flora, and leave your intestines completely sterile and incapable of healthful digestion.

- **Overly sterilized environment.** Protecting yourself from bacteria can prevent illness, but living in an overly sterilized environment full of antibacterial sprays and soaps can also deprive your body of the exposure to bacteria that it was designed to expect. This **hygiene hypothesis,** first published in the *British Medical Journal* in 1989, has garnered a lot of mainstream attention recently and attributes many disorders—such as eczema, multiple sclerosis, inflammatory bowel disease (IBD), and other autoimmune disorders—to a lack of interaction with bacteria.

> ***Hygiene hypothesis:***
> *A recently popularized hypothesis that states a lack of exposure to infectious agents, symbiotic microorganisms, and parasites increases susceptibility to allergic diseases by hampering immune-system development.*

If you try your best to avoid the pitfalls listed above, you can succeed at lessening the impact of dysbacteriosis on your health and digestion. However, I firmly believe that **in our modern environment, it is almost impossible to maintain a low-carb lifestyle without first regrowing this lost organ of microflora.**

This is why so many people who started on other low-carb diets gave up once constipation related to a sterile gut set in. In fact, constipation is the number one reason for failure on low-carb diets, because it seems to reinforce the age-old and incorrect belief that fiber from grains is absolutely vital to digestion. If that sounds similar to your own experience, know that you actually have nothing to worry about.

Probiotics:
Supplements that restore your gut flora and healthy digestion by delivering micro-organisms to the intestines. If your flora is damaged or missing, these supplements are essential for restoring balance to your body and for losing weight.

Since the low-carb craze of previous years has come and gone, a new and vital supplement has begun to enter the mainstream conversation about optimal health. This new supplement fixes the broken link in the low-carb chain, and is a vital element of the Belly Fat Cure—it will ensure not only an accelerated transformation in just 14 days, but the **consistent weight-loss results no other program can deliver.**

Probiotics

You have probably already heard some good things about **probiotics,** since they have a fairly sterling reputation. However, few people seem to be talking about just how important this simple supplement is. That is a shame, because of this fact:

**It is extremely difficult
to reach your goal weight
or desired level of health without repairing
your gut flora with a probiotic supplement first.**

Most likely you turned to some überfibrous cereal, bread, or supplement the moment you perceived yourself to be constipated, and have been an enthusiastic member of the "fiber fan club" ever since. That's nothing to feel bad about, because I used to feel the same way.

A probiotic treats the cause of your constipation, dysbacteriosis, rather than sweeping it under the rug the way laxatives and too much fiber do. It is also free of side effects, bringing you the following benefits instead:

1. Bacteria in the gut create all sorts of essential vitamins, including vitamins B_{12} and K.

2. Intestinal flora help regulate inflammation and immune-system response, as well as protect against the development of inflammatory diseases.

You can order the probiotic I trust the most, Primal Flora™, at **TheBellyFatCure.com**. This product is made by Mark Sisson, author of *The Primal Blueprint,* whom I consider to be the most forward-thinking creator of nutritional products in the country. I personally take one each and every day for good measure, but it is only necessary that you take them long enough to repair and restore your flora, or after intestinal trauma such as diarrhea or a course of antibiotics.

I talk a lot about making this program easier by using mostly foods that you can find anywhere, and fortunately we live in a time where probiotics are on sale in more stores than ever before. If you prefer not to order probiotics online, your local drugstore or health-food store should have several options. If you only have access to conventional grocery stores, ask them to carry a probiotic . . . you may be surprised to find out that they already do! Just be wary of any yogurts or other products that claim to offer the benefits of probiotics, as many are packed full of hidden sugar.

The bottom line of the fiber myth is this: we have been trying to replace the many functions of the over 500 species of living bacteria in our body with dead fiber from the least ideal sources, and the results have been extremely disappointing. Only when we cut through the marketing claims to discover better fiber, and use this better fiber in conjunction with healthy gut flora, can we expect to approach optimal digestion and the accelerated weight loss that comes with it. Health and beauty will come to you if you nurture them from the inside out!

Digestion Perfection Checklist

If you're having trouble with digestion, follow these steps, in this order:

1. **Probiotic supplement:** Take 2 to 3 servings of a probiotic daily. It should be in a capsule, have 30 billion or more cultures, and contain multiple strains of bacteria.

2. **Super Carbs:** Increase your intake of high-fiber Super Carbs, especially artichoke hearts, broccoli, brussels sprouts, and collard greens. Nuts are also an excellent source of fiber.

3. **Fiber supplement:** Take 1 to 2 servings of a *soluble* fiber supplement each day. Check the label to ensure it is free of sugar and artificial flavorings. For a list of the soluble fiber supplements my clients like best, please visit **TheBellyFatCure.com**.

4. **Salt balance:** Drink 1 to 2 cups of chicken stock or chicken broth before bed. This may correct a salt imbalance in the body that is preventing smooth movements.

5. **Magnesium:** Some clients experienced improved digestion after adding 1 serving of a magnesium supplement to their bedtime routine. Magnesium has additional bone-health benefits.

You can use one, none, or all of these strategies—although I do recommend attempting them in the order listed. I do not recommend laxatives of any kind.

Are You Ready to Transform?

Again, before you can be ready for your two-week transformation on the Fast Track, you must release all the following myths:

1. The myth that calories control your fat tissue

2. The myth that grains and starches help all people lose weight

3. The myth that digestion requires "high-fiber food *products*"

If you have committed to throwing out these core obstacles that Conventional Wisdom, Inc., has used to keep you in a vicious cycle of endless dieting, you are ready to get going and begin your two-week transformation . . . starting today!

FAST TRACK
SUCCESS
STORY

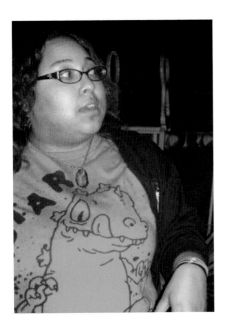

Before

Age: 21
Height: 5'6"
Pounds Lost: 44

Like a lot of girls I know, I gained weight after graduating from high school. Unfortunately, it wasn't 5 or 10 pounds . . . it was *50* pounds in only a few short years. All that weight made me feel trapped because I knew I didn't want to spend my entire adult life being overweight and unhealthy. That is how I felt on the day when I just happened to see Jorge on TV asking for volunteers to try his new Fast Track edition of the Belly Fat Cure.

When I first started, I was as skeptical as anyone else. Everything I had been told about eating healthy and losing weight seemed to be contradicted by what Jorge was saying . . . so much so that I left our first meeting worried that I would gain weight if I stuck to the Fast Track Menu. But when I stepped on the scale after that first week and saw that I'd lost 12 pounds, I was an immediate believer! I felt as if I had eaten more food that week than any other week but still lost weight, which seemed crazy—I had always thought the only way to lose weight was to go hungry.

Since Day 1, I've experienced nothing but continual results without ever feeling hungry. I can honestly say that deciding to give Jorge's advice a try was one of the best decisions I've ever made. Jorge took a lot of knowledge that I would have found frustrating and confusing and turned it into something fun and easy for me to understand.

I used to either not care or simply not know the impact that food would have on my body, but now I know exactly how each bite I take

Catherine
Lost 44 pounds!

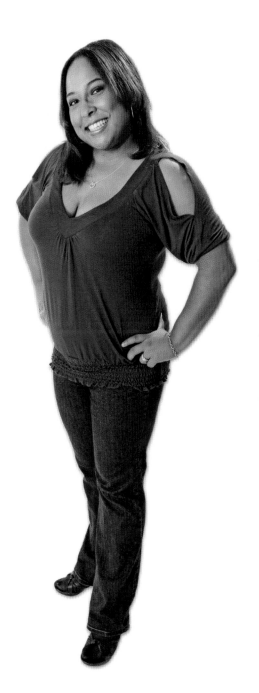

moves me closer to my goal weight. Other than all the weight I've lost, my favorite thing about this program is that I feel so knowledgeable about nutrition! It's a really empowering feeling.

What's Next?

I've lost all the weight I put on after high school, but now I have new goals I never even dreamed of. I used to think that I had no choice about being overweight because it was just part of my genetics. Now I know that it's not about genetics, but habits. That means no more excuses! I haven't stopped losing weight yet, and I'm gonna keep going. . . .

My Best Tip

Follow the program to the letter! As I said, I was super nervous when I first saw the foods on the Fast Track Menu. I thought about changing a few things—removing yolks, getting low-fat this or that—but I didn't. I decided I would follow it 100 percent, exactly as is, and just move on when it didn't work. But guess what? It worked!

FAST TRACK
SUCCESS
STORY

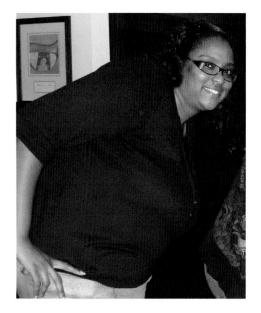

Before

Age: 35
Height: 5'10"
Pounds Lost: 30

This is, hands down, the best weight-loss experience of my life—and I know a thing or seven about diets! My favorite benefit is that I have more energy than I can ever remember. I used to drag my tired self out of bed every morning at 5:30 to let my dog out, but now I am literally leaping out of bed with a sense of excitement to start the day. I don't just let my dog out anymore either; I actually enjoy taking him for a walk. I think he must still be adjusting because he looks at me like I'm crazy for being so awake that early!

For the first time, I am confident in my ability to stick to a plan that will give me health and energy for the rest of my life, because it really is that easy. I am a veteran dieter who has tried everything, only to lose then gain then lose then gain some more . . . so a weight-loss program that actually inspires confidence is totally foreign to me. After so many diets that broke me down, I can't believe someone figured out how to create a program that builds me up and still works.

What's Next?

My outlook on life is so much brighter, and feeling like every day is going to be my best is just invaluable yet almost indescribable. I have

Vinneeca
Lost 30 pounds!

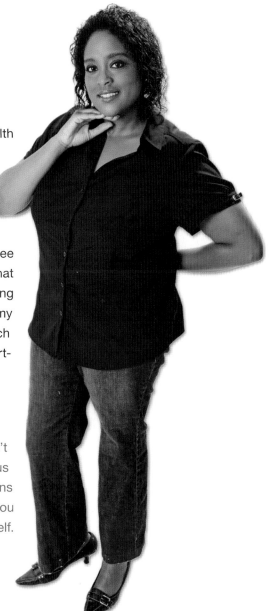

so many new goals now that I feel my health is on track, most of which include helping family and friends who are also struggling with weight. I'm so passionate about the Belly Fat Cure when I'm telling family members what they need to do to feel better and lose weight, and I can see in their eyes how proud they are of me. That makes me feel great, but so will accomplishing one of my final personal goals: I'm working my way toward buying a ticket to a tropical beach where I can wear a swimsuit and be comfortable . . . for the first time in my life!

My Best Tip

Stop thinking in terms of what you can't have and start thinking about all the delicious food you *can* have! This simple switch turns that old diet mentality off, which means you are so much less likely to give up on yourself. You're worth it!

FAST TRACK
SUCCESS
STORY

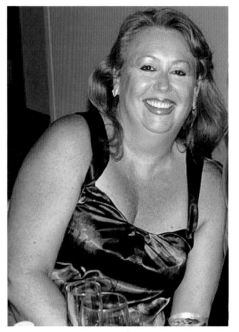

Before

Age: 50

Height: 5'9"

Pounds Lost: 70

Before starting on the Fast Track program, I felt like I was just waiting. I was ready to lose weight, I wanted to lose weight, but I was still just . . . waiting! Luckily, a very good friend put me in touch with Jorge at the start of his BFC Fast Track program, and I just knew that this was the moment I had been waiting for.

Life since I started has been totally amazing! I am sugar free, healthy, strong, empowered, and confident. I can now make truly healthy choices, because Jorge has opened up my eyes to all the traps out there designed to trick people who are trying their best to make the right choices. And for the first time ever, I can finally say "No" to the foods I thought I depended on, because I realize just how great life can be without them.

It has also been amazing to be able to help other people I care about who want to lose weight. Once the first 10 pounds came off, a few of my co-workers started asking for my secrets—and now that I've lost 70, they all want to know what I'm eating! Jorge's program and philosophy are so simple that it's easy to help others who have questions about how to get healthier . . . and helping others feels just as great as losing weight. Well, almost!

Debra
Lost 70 pounds!

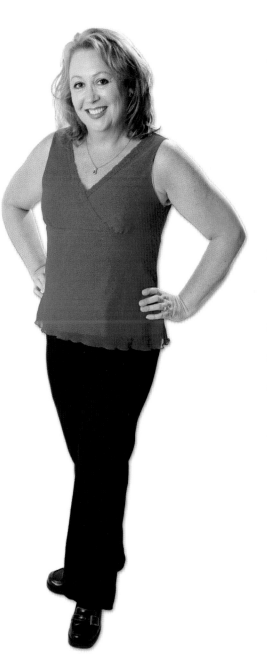

What's Next?

When you rediscover the confidence you thought you had lost, everything changes. I'm not just more confident in how I look and feel, I'm confident because I achieved my goal. The program is great—but at the end of the day, I'm the one who made the right choices, did the right things, and made the weight disappear. Knowing that I can accomplish anything I set my mind to has opened up so many new doors to explore in my life. Who knows where they will lead?!

My Best Tip

Be prepared! Always have a snack with you (in your purse or the refrigerator) so that you can reach for a good choice. Having string cheese and cucumber slices in my fridge has saved me many times!

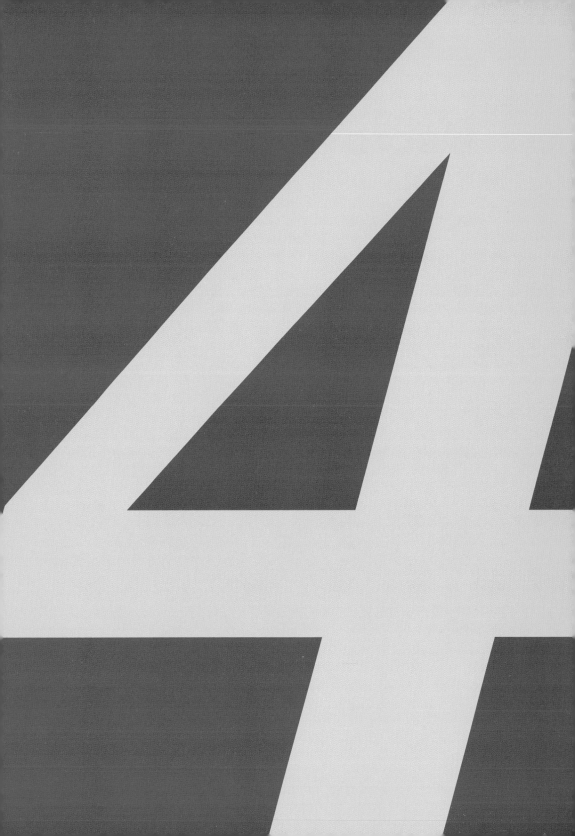

The 14-Day Challenge
and Beyond

"Simplicity is the ultimate sophistication."

— **LEONARDO DA VINCI**

The Belly Fat Cure Fast Track program is not another fad diet. It works great to supercharge the Belly Fat Cure for 14 days, but it can also be used as a life-style plan that will guide you to fuel your body with the nutri-ents it was designed to thrive on beyond just two weeks. If you stick to the simple yet so-phisticated **Fast Track Menu** to satisfy your physical hunger, you will experience an almost im-mediate cascade of health benefits . . . the most noticeable being *dramatic* weight loss.

> *Fast Track Menu:*
> The simplest and most delicious menu of nutritious foods that keep your belly fat loss at the maximum.

Your 14-Day Challenge

If you follow the Fast Track Menu exactly, as my most success-ful clients have done, you will come as close to losing 14 pounds in 14 days as is possible for your own body. As an added bonus, you'll also experience a complete transformation of your energy levels, hunger, hormones, and digestion—all of which will vastly improve your quality of life, regardless of whether you lose 14 pounds or 4. When it comes to tracking numerical weight loss, the bottom line is this: every ounce counts! Every ounce of belly fat lost, no matter how slowly, benefits you and the people who love you. So stop stressing and start celebrating!

For right now, all you need to do is commit to two weeks on this advanced edition of the Belly Fat Cure. However, you must commit *fully* during these two weeks. No slips, no cheats, no excuses . . . but try it for just two weeks! I want you to stay motivated with the knowledge that not only will many of the meals be ready in minutes, but they will all taste super good as well. I personally created the menus to make sure that you say "Yummy!" every day for those two weeks (especially at night). You will have all the freedom to add more variety back into your diet once you have mastered the basics of this program and brought balance to your sweet tooth.

What you eat or don't eat will always be your choice. My job is to simply show you which foods will signal your body to shed fat and produce health, and try to explain as clearly as I can why these foods work the way they do. Whether you continue on with the Fast Track Menu after 14 days and explore your Fast Track options with the Belly Best Foods list, or transition to the original Belly Fat Cure program, is up to you. Many of my clients return to tracking 15 grams of sugar and 6 servings of carbs after they complete their 14-day challenge, while others follow the Fast Track program for a longer period of time. Before you can make your decision, you must witness the astounding results with your very own eyes.

First and foremost, I think it will be very helpful for you to fill out the following contract. Post it where you can see it, as a sign of your commitment to this program and to yourself:

The BELLY FAT CURE™

FAST TRACK
Success Contract

I, _____, commit to following the Fast Track Menu and the principles of the Fast Track exactly for just 14 days, because my body and my life are worth it.

Regardless of all else, I am committed to loving myself and my body, and to releasing the need for validation from others. Everything I need in order to be happy is already in my heart, and I will remember that not only for 14 days, but for the rest of my life.

Signature _____

I currently weigh _____

My favorite quality about myself is _____

I'd love to see this number on the scale _____

I'll reward myself with _____

Someone else I'd like to help become healthier is _____

_____

When You're Ready to Get Started

As your coach, here is the number one method I recommend to get the best results on the Fast Track: Follow the 14-Day Fast Track Menu to the letter, with no changes. Zip. Nada. Follow the plan. The Fast Track Menu is a simple and tasty way to avoid confusion and build momentum instantly. Thousands of my clients have achieved great success by following this menu exactly. I highly recommend you model their success.

Okay, I can hear some of you right now, "Can I *please* change something?" My answer: please refer to above paragraph. "But, *Jorge* . . . " All right, let's talk about this. First, let me once more emphasize the value in following the menu as you get started: it's delicious and economical, and it keeps you on track for optimal heath and belly fat loss. Second, yes, I did design the Fast Track Menu to have flexibility for various reasons—including dietary restrictions. So if you truly feel the need to make adjustments, there are six important guidelines to follow:

1. An entire day's menu can be repeated exactly every day for the entire two weeks. For example, if variety is not the spice of your life and Day 3 reads like poetry to your senses, then repeat Day 3 for Days 1 though 14.

2. A meal or snack can be exchanged for another meal or snack within its *category* from any day on the Fast Track Menu. For example, if dinner from Day 2 was incredible, and you're ready to enjoy it for dinner again on Day 4 . . . you can! In the same way, a lunch can be exchanged for another lunch, and a snack for another snack.

3. An item within a meal can be exchanged with another item from its category. Proteins can be exchanged for proteins, Super Carbs for Super Carbs, and so on. If the protein for dinner is salmon, but your taste buds are calling for sautéed chicken breast, feel free to go with the chicken instead. Or if asparagus is the chosen Super Carb, but you're more of a mushrooms and broccoli type of person, go ahead! I've provided a categorized Belly Best Foods list in Chapter 6 with all your Fast Track Menu foods options.

4. The Fast Track Menu is all about easy, tossed-together meals. If, however, you love spending time in the kitchen and take joy in your culinary creations, Chapter 5 is for you. I've given you many tasty Ultimate Carb Swap recipe options for all parts of your day: breakfast, lunch, dinner, snacks, and treats. It is important to substitute these recipes only for similar meals or snacks. For example, my famous Chocolate Lace Cookies are perfect for an evening treat, and my mouthwatering Steak Béarnaise is a great choice for dinner.

5. For those of you constantly on the go, I recommend substituting meals with a stevia-sweetened whey protein shake. Each shake should have at least 20 grams of protein and be very low in sugar (I recommend Jay Robb or Primal Fuel brands—you can find out more about these products at: **TheBellyFatCure.com**).

6. Your treat is something to delight in every evening, so here are some substitutions to savor: In place of dark chocolate, bake a batch of my Chocolate Lace Cookies, and enjoy two each night with your hot beverage. Or relax with two glasses of red wine or two vodka/club sodas as a substitute to your sweet treat and hot beverage. You may also substitute one serving of fruit as your evening treat (please see page 161 for portion size).

FAST TRACK MENU
Day 1

BREAKFAST

2 eggs, fried

Bacon

Cheese

Coffee with half-and-half

SNACK

Pecans (¼ cup)

LUNCH

Spinach salad

Chicken breast

Bell peppers

Olive oil-and-vinegar dressing

SNACK

Deli meat (1 serving)

DINNER

Grilled salmon

Asparagus

Salt and pepper, to taste

TREAT

Dark chocolate (85%, up to 1 oz.)

Hot beverage with low-sugar whipped cream

FAST TRACK MENU
Day 2

BREAKFAST

2 eggs, scrambled

Avocado

Mushrooms

Coffee with half-and-half

SNACK

Cheese (1 serving)

LUNCH

Lettuce-wrapped hamburger patty

Avocado

Cucumbers

SNACK

Hard-boiled egg

DINNER

Sautéed pork chops

Broccoli

Mushrooms

Salt and pepper, to taste

TREAT

Dark chocolate (85%, up to 1 oz.)

Hot beverage with low-sugar whipped cream

FAST TRACK MENU
Day 3

BREAKFAST

Cottage cheese

Walnuts

Coffee with half-and-half

SNACK

Almonds (¼ cup)

LUNCH

Sautéed chicken breast

Bell peppers

Broccoli

SNACK

Cheese (1 serving)

DINNER

Sautéed steak

Brussels sprouts

Mushrooms

Salt and pepper, to taste

TREAT

Dark chocolate (85%, up to 1 oz.)

Hot beverage with low-sugar whipped cream

FAST TRACK MENU
Day 4

BREAKFAST

2 eggs, sunny-side up

Bacon

Coffee with half-and-half

SNACK

Deli meat (1 serving)

LUNCH

Tuna

Avocado

Mixed greens

SNACK

Macadamia nuts (12 raw)

DINNER

Sautéed tilapia

Artichoke

Cauliflower

Salt and pepper, to taste

TREAT

Dark chocolate (85%, up to 1 oz.)

Hot beverage with low-sugar whipped cream

FAST TRACK MENU
Day 5

BREAKFAST

3-egg omelette
Avocado
Mushrooms
Cheese
Coffee with half-and-half

SNACK

Walnuts (¼ cup)

LUNCH

Mixed-greens salad
Chicken breast
Artichoke
Cheese
Olive oil-and-vinegar dressing

SNACK

Cheese (1 serving)

DINNER

Sautéed halibut
Spinach
Bell peppers
Salt and pepper, to taste

TREAT

Dark chocolate (85%, up to 1 oz.)

Hot beverage with low-sugar whipped cream

FAST TRACK MENU
Day 6

BREAKFAST

Cottage cheese

Walnuts

Coffee with half-and-half

SNACK

Pumpkin seeds (¼ cup)

LUNCH

Sautéed chicken breast

Asparagus

Salt and pepper, to taste

SNACK

Deli meat (1 serving)

DINNER

Sautéed pork chops

Broccoli

Mushrooms

Salt and pepper, to taste

TREAT

Dark chocolate (85%, up to 1 oz.)

Hot beverage with low-sugar whipped cream

FAST TRACK MENU
Day 7

BREAKFAST

2-egg omelette

Sausage

Avocado

Coffee with half-and-half

SNACK

Hard-boiled egg

LUNCH

Grilled hamburger patty

Cheese

Cucumbers

SNACK

Cheese (1 serving)

DINNER

Grilled salmon

Spinach

Salt and pepper, to taste

TREAT

Dark chocolate (85%, up to 1 oz.)

Hot beverage with low-sugar whipped cream

FAST TRACK MENU
Day 8

BREAKFAST

3-egg omelette
Avocado
Mushrooms
Cheese
Coffee with half-and-half

SNACK

Macadamia nuts (12 raw)

LUNCH

Tuna
Sautéed asparagus
Salt and pepper, to taste

SNACK

Deli meat (1 serving)

DINNER

Sautéed steak
Brussels sprouts
Mushrooms
Salt and pepper, to taste

TREAT

Dark chocolate (85%, up to 1 oz.)

Hot beverage with low-sugar whipped cream

FAST TRACK MENU
Day 9

BREAKFAST

2 eggs, fried
Bacon
Cheese
Coffee with half-and-half

SNACK

Cheese (1 serving)

LUNCH

Mixed-greens salad
Chicken breast
Artichoke
Cheese
Olive oil-and-vinegar dressing

SNACK

Almonds (¼ cup)

DINNER

Grilled halibut
Cauliflower
Zucchini
Salt and pepper, to taste

TREAT

Dark chocolate (85%, up to 1 oz.)
Hot beverage with low-sugar whipped cream

FAST TRACK MENU
Day 10

BREAKFAST

Cottage cheese

Walnuts

Coffee with half-and-half

SNACK

Deli meat (1 serving)

LUNCH

Tuna

Avocado

Mixed greens

Olive oil-and-vinegar dressing

SNACK

Macadamia nuts (12 raw)

DINNER

Grilled pork chops

Broccoli

Mushrooms

Salt and pepper, to taste

TREAT

Dark chocolate (85%, up to 1 oz.)

Hot beverage with low-sugar whipped cream

FAST TRACK MENU
Day 11

BREAKFAST

2 eggs, fried
Bacon
Cheese
Coffee with half-and-half

SNACK

Deli meat (1 serving)

LUNCH

Lettuce-wrapped hamburger patty
Avocado
Cucumbers

SNACK

Pumpkin seeds (¼ cup)

DINNER

Sautéed halibut
Spinach
Bell peppers
Salt and pepper, to taste

TREAT

Dark chocolate (85%, up to 1 oz.)

Hot beverage with low-sugar whipped cream

FAST TRACK MENU
Day 12

BREAKFAST

Cottage cheese
Walnuts
Coffee with half-and-half

SNACK

Cheese (1 serving)

LUNCH

Mixed-greens salad
Chicken breast
Artichoke
Cheese
Olive oil-and-vinegar dressing

SNACK

Sunflower seeds (¼ cup)

DINNER

Grilled pork chop
Squash
Salt and pepper, to taste

TREAT

Dark chocolate (85%, up to 1 oz.)

Hot beverage with low-sugar whipped cream

FAST TRACK MENU
Day 13

BREAKFAST

3-egg omelette
Avocado
Mushrooms
Cheese
Coffee with half-and-half

SNACK

Macadamia nuts (12 raw)

LUNCH

Lettuce-wrapped hamburger patty
Cheese
Avocado
Bacon

SNACK

Hard-boiled egg

DINNER

Grilled salmon
Asparagus
Zucchini
Salt and pepper, to taste

TREAT

Dark chocolate (85%, up to 1 oz.)

Hot beverage with low-sugar whipped cream

FAST TRACK MENU
Day 14

BREAKFAST

2 eggs, scrambled
Bacon
Cheese
Coffee with half-and-half

SNACK

Brazil nuts (¼ cup)

LUNCH

Romaine salad
Chicken breast
Artichoke
Olive oil-and-vinegar dressing

SNACK

Cheese (1 serving)

DINNER

Sautéed steak
Brussels sprouts
Mushrooms
Salt and pepper, to taste

TREAT

Dark chocolate (85%, up to 1 oz.)
Hot beverage with low-sugar whipped cream

Tips for Food Preparation

1. Fry those eggs! You'll notice that many of your mornings start with eggs for breakfast. Prepare them any way you want: scrambled; poached; and, yes, fried. My favorite oils for cooking are olive and coconut, but you can use PAM Olive Oil or butter as well. Just don't use the whole can of PAM Olive Oil or half a stick of butter.

2. Avoid canola oil and margarine. While I'm open to most preparation methods, I absolutely recommend steering clear of canola oil at all costs. Margarine is also a big "no-no" since it is hydrogenated and heavily processed.

Approved Drinks

1. Coffee with heavy cream or half-and-half. Do not use milk (nonfat, reduced fat, or whole). Sweeten if desired with one of the following approved sweeteners: xylitol, erythritol, or plain stevia. Limit 2 per day.

2. Tea, hot or iced. You may use an approved sweetener, or lemon and lime. Limit 2 per day for dark teas; green tea is allowed in unlimited amounts.

3. Water, flat or sparkling. You may use lemon and lime.

Quick Guidelines for Your 14-Day Challenge

- Before starting, take your preliminary waist measurement. Suck in your stomach and measure around your belly button. To determine your maximum healthy waist measurement, take your height and divide it in half. I am 6' tall (72") so I am aiming for a waist measurement of less than 36". Go to **TheBellyFatCure .com** to watch Dr. Oz demonstrate exactly how to obtain an accurate measure.

- Understand that no item on the menu is allowed in "unlimited" amounts, as even healthy foods need to be eaten in moderation.

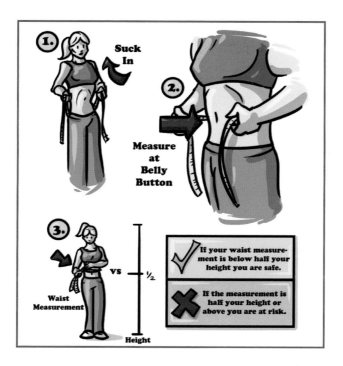

- For those foods listed that do not have a serving size indicated, consider an amount equal to the size of your palm as a serving; eat no more than 2 servings of any one item in a sitting. Also, a palm-size serving and a heaping handful are not the same thing!

- Try to drink 6 to 8 glasses of water per day (48 to 64 oz.), but also allow your urine to guide you. If you need to urinate every 20 minutes, you may be over-hydrated. If it is dark in color and/or cloudy, you are dehydrated. Balance your hydration according to your thirst and the appearance of your urine, taking comfort in the fact that the foods I recommend are made mostly of water!

- Protein and meal-replacement shakes can be mixed in water, unsweetened almond milk, unsweetened coconut milk, or unsweetened hemp milk. Blender Ball bottles are inexpensive and make blending shakes quick, easy, and clean.

- If you experience difficulty moving your bowels, please see my "Digestion Perfection Checklist" on page 56. You can also print a copy of this checklist at **TheBellyFatCure.com**.

- Ask yourself, "Am I hungry for the next bite?" about halfway through each meal. As soon as you're no longer physically hungry for the next bite, wrap up the leftovers and save them for later.

- If you feel "full," you have overeaten!

- Yes, you may skip snacks or even meals if you're not physically hungry.

- *Never* skip a snack or a meal if you *do* feel physically hungry.

- Dressings and sauces can make or break your weight loss. For the first 14 days, simply mix three parts extra-virgin olive oil with one part red wine or apple cider vinegar for a tangy and versatile Greek-style dressing.

- If you'd like to have both chocolate and wine as your treat, I recommend 1 glass of red wine with 1 serving (2.5 sugar grams or less) of dark chocolate.

- For adult treats, you may have other *sugar-free* alcohol (white wine, tequila, and so forth), but I do not recommend them. My clients experience the best results when they limit their adult treat to red wine or vodka. Beer is not approved while on the Fast Track program.

- When you feel hungry between meals, having a **snack** is helpful as a source of energy and nutrients to get you safely from one meal to the next, without falling victim to some food that will reverse your weight loss. Snacking on good fats and what I call **Restorative Proteins**™ will ease the transition to your new metabolism.

- Neither sweet **treats** nor alcohol will help you lose weight, but they may very well keep you sane and satisfied. The sweet treats I recommend, when eaten in moderation, are the smartest way to satisfy your sweet tooth with as little impact on your weight loss as possible. If you do not have cravings for these treats and drinks, simply skip these options and your weight loss will be accelerated.

- When an option is listed as **ideal** (uncured, organic, and the like), for optimal health you should choose that option whenever it is available to you. If the ideal option is not available, you may choose a conventional option and your weight loss will not be compromised. The best example of this is bacon: while it is one of my favorite foods, it can be overly processed and contain nitrates and other preservatives that aren't ideal for total health. Look for uncured, less-processed bacon whenever it is available, but know that even processed bacon is better for weight loss than sugars and starches.

I'd again like to offer my encouragement in sticking to the program through the first 14 days, because the payoff is tremendous. If you're like most people, you may experience cravings for sugar, grains, and starches as your fat-*storing* metabolism dies and your new fat-*burning* metabolism replaces it. Patience is crucial here; most likely you've been riding a blood-sugar roller coaster for years now, and it will take a minimum of two weeks to bring balance and your new metabolism to life.

Snack:
A source of energy and nutrients that is designed to get you safely from one meal to the next, without falling victim to some food that will reverse your weight loss.

Restorative Proteins:
Natural protein from animals and plants that repairs and replaces damaged tissue in your body.

Treats:
Foods that will not directly help you lose weight, but may keep you sane and on course while satisfying your sweet tooth.

Ideal:
An option that is most beneficial to your weight loss and overall health, but not essential if it is unavailable or unaffordable.

How Much Water?

We've been taught that we need at least eight glasses of water per day, but what has been lost in that message is that we actually get a significant amount of water from our food if we're eating properly. In fact, one daily requirement for water cannot be generalized for everyone, as variations in size, activity level, diet, and even geography impact each individual's needs.

Drinking too much water can, in fact, have a negative effect on your electrolytes, so you must learn to allow your thirst as well as the volume and color of your urine to determine the amount of water that is right for you. As I said earlier in the chapter, if your urine is absolutely clear and you're running to the bathroom every 20 minutes, you're drinking too much water. If it's dark or cloudy, you're not drinking enough. (Note: eight glasses each day may be too much.)

Day 15 and Beyond

After you complete the 14-day challenge, there are two options to continue losing belly fat. I recommend them in the following order:

1. Keep using the Fast Track Menu, Ultimate Carb Swap Recipes, and Belly Best Foods list. Again, I find it effective to provide my clients with a simple structure. The Fast Track Menu is your safety net . . . simple, economical, and effective. Additionally, I always find that my most successful clients automate the majority of their meals. I highly recommend that you model their success.

> **Belly Best Foods:**
> The Fast Track foods that keep glucagon levels exceptionally high by keeping insulin low.

Automation aside, what makes the Fast Track a functional and flavorful lifestyle are hundreds of options to eat healthfully while celebrating your love for food. Think of creating delicious and fast meals from the Fast Track Menu as time well spent as you perfect your mastery of fat-melting foods. Beyond this menu, The Belly Best Foods list has all the elements you need to create your own custom-designed energizing lifestyle—you're free to dabble in any of the thousands of delicious combinations and further hone your creativity.

2. Transition to the original Belly Fat Cure program. The success my clients continue to experience through the Fast Track is astonishing. I will admit, however, as effective as this program is at burning belly fat, it can be a challenging lifestyle to adopt. If, after your 14-day challenge, you want to transition to the original Belly Fat Cure program, that's okay! I encourage you to choose the program that is best for both your lifestyle and weight-loss goals. Both programs allow you to eat healthfully, without trading in your sanity or your love of food.

Healthy goal weight:
A weight and body composition at which you're both comfortable in your clothes and optimally healthy. Because of the body images we're exposed to daily, many people mistake a healthy goal weight for being "fat."

Energy:
The power that we obtain from food and convert into movement, functions, and thoughts.

Still Not Losing?

If you tried going back to the menu but cannot lose weight, even by sticking to it exactly, then you may have reached the all-too-familiar weight-loss plateau. Typically, most people can hit their **healthy goal weight** without running into a plateau. Others, however, require a little extra effort and planning to accelerate fat loss or to reach a competition weight; that is, a weight and body composition that is closer to that of an athlete, and closer to the images we see in magazines. (Note that while it's always great to work toward a motivating goal, competition weight is no healthier than a healthy goal weight. In fact, striving for an unrealistic competition weight may do more harm than good.)

It is at the point of reaching a plateau—only after your hormones have been balanced, your flora has been restored, and your metabolism has transformed to one that burns rather than stores fat—that it becomes time to consider one final weight-loss element: **energy.**

Breaking the Plateau

Let me be very clear about one thing: I always tell people, "The Belly Fat Cure isn't about eating less and exercising more." And it still isn't, even when you're on the Fast Track. You see, Conventional Wisdom, Inc., has put calories and exercise at the top of the weight-loss checklist, and that fact is the main reason our country is fat and sick . . . our focus on *how many* calories instead of *what kind* of calories is literally killing us.

Energy deficit:
A state of expending more energy that you consume. Only after hormonal balance has been achieved and a fat-burning metabolism has been created does encouraging an energy deficit become a helpful weight-loss tool. Focusing purely on the energy deficit—as Conventional Wisdom, Inc., suggests—leads to dieting, hunger, and failure.

With the Belly Fat Cure, encouraging an **energy deficit** is that last step on the road to a healthy weight. Expending more energy than you consume is meaningless and ineffective in the long term when you're riding up and down a toxic sugar spiral, laying the foundation for chronic disease and consistently storing body fat despite your most valiant efforts. It's called context, and when the facts regarding calories and exercise are put into context with the science of insulin and metabolism, you begin to realize just how wrong so many people have been about weight loss for all these years.

So, what are my recommendations for when you need to break through a plateau? Try them one at a time, in this order:

1. Increase your **play** (any activity that requires any kind of movement and optional smiling). Most people are naturally more active at this point due to the increased energy the Fast Track plan brings and won't need to make a conscious effort to exercise.

2. Cut back on—or skip altogether—the sweet treats and adult treats.

3. Incorporate my optional exercise recommendations from Chapter 8 into your routine.

The great thing about the preceding three recommendations is that, with your old sugar and starch metabolism, they would have seemed impossible. *Consistent energy to play? Control over my cravings? No way!* But now that your body is supplied by an even stream of energy thanks to the power of good fats, and every cell is reinvigorated with the nutrients from Super Carbs, you will absolutely crave movement! Your body is awake now, and it's itching to go outside and play! Also, thanks to good fats and Restorative Proteins, your hunger is satiated for long periods of time, banishing uncontrollable cravings for quick fixes of inferior fuel.

I'm still not advising you to waste your time counting a single calorie . . . I'd much rather you walk your dog farther or play with your kids more often. If that doesn't work, try cutting back on the size and frequency of sweet treats. If you want to improve your heart health, tone your body, and increase fat loss, enjoy the gym-free walking and strength exercises I lay out in Chapter 8. If you put a little more energy into the universe and consume just a little less energy from treats, you will destroy any plateau that gets in your way . . . and still not feel hungry or deprived.

These are the final, and least influential, steps to reaching either a healthy goal weight or a competition weight. **It should come as no surprise that by treating deprivation and exhaustion as the gold standards of weight loss, so many honest people continue to fail.** It is unfortunate that the deck is stacked against the truth . . . the status quo has nothing to gain and everything to lose if people know the truth.

That is why I need you. It is going to require ordinary people who experience the benefits firsthand to spread this truth to our families and loved ones. It is vital that you and others like you become ambassadors of health, motivated not by profit but by a desire to help others. Only then can our generation seize this monumental tipping point and reverse the rising tide of disease that threatens us all.

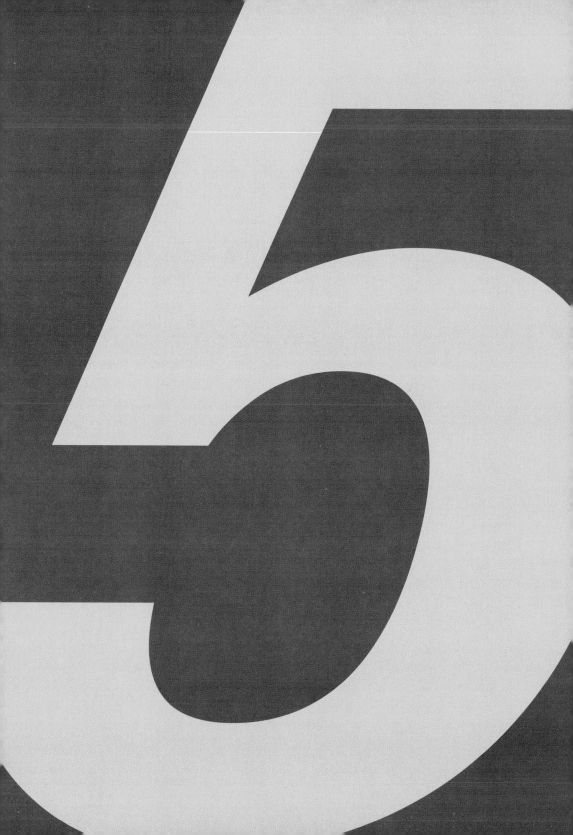

Ultimate
Carb Swap
Recipes

"The world is but canvas to our imaginations."

— **HENRY DAVID THOREAU**

The recipes in this chapter are for those of you I described at the beginning of Chapter 4: at-home chefs who thrive on creativity in the kitchen. As always, my recommendation is to follow the Fast Track Menu exactly, with no changes. However, when you're ready to venture outside the basic meals of the Menu, I've included many of my favorite Ultimate Carb Swap recipes in this chapter. Remember to only substitute a recipe with a like meal or snack, and to use the Fast Track Menu as your guide. If you love these recipes, check out **TheBellyFatCure.com** for more.

Bon appétit!

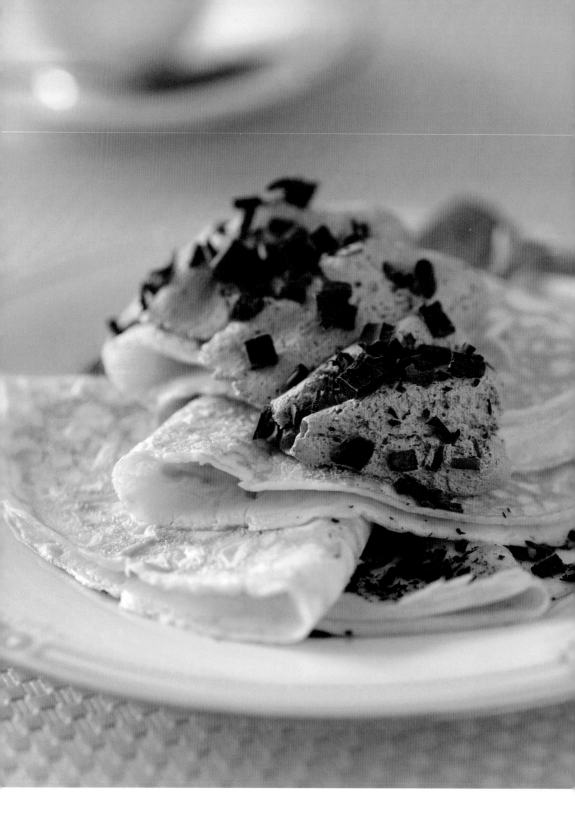

BELLY FAT CURE SWEET CHOCOLATE MOUSSE CRÊPES

Delicious chocolate mousse served with sweet crêpes, whipped cream, and grated dark chocolate.

MAKES 4 SERVINGS

For Sweet Crêpes:

4 large eggs
2 Tbsp. cream
½ tsp. salt
½ tsp. vanilla extract
Butter

For Chocolate Mousse:

½ pint cold low-sugar whipping cream
1 tsp. vanilla extract
4 oz. dark chocolate (85% or greater),
    finely chopped
8 oz. cream cheese, softened
½ cup sour cream
1 tsp. instant espresso powder

If you would like the crêpes a little sweeter, add 1 tsp. xylitol.
If you would like the chocolate mousse a little sweeter, add 2 Tbsp. xylitol.

For crêpes: Whisk together eggs, cream, salt, and vanilla extract (and xylitol, if you like) in a small mixing bowl until thoroughly blended.

Heat an omelette pan over medium to medium-high heat. Lightly coat the bottom and sides of the pan with butter. Ladle a small amount of batter in the pan; about 2½ Tbsp. Tip the pan back and forth to thinly coat the bottom of the pan. Cook until set, and then lift and flip the crêpe, being careful not to tear it. Cook 1 minute more. Slide crêpe out of pan and onto a dish. Continue making crêpes until all of the batter is gone.

For mousse: In small mixing bowl, beat cream and vanilla together on high speed until almost stiff.

Melt chocolate in the microwave in 15-second intervals, stirring after each, until melted.

In a medium mixing bowl, beat softened cream cheese (and xylitol, if you like) for 3 minutes. Beat in sour cream and espresso powder. Add melted chocolate and beat until combined.

Fold in a third of the whipped cream with a rubber spatula. Gently fold in remaining whipped cream until just combined. Spoon into crêpes or pipe on top of crêpes and garnish with grated dark chocolate.

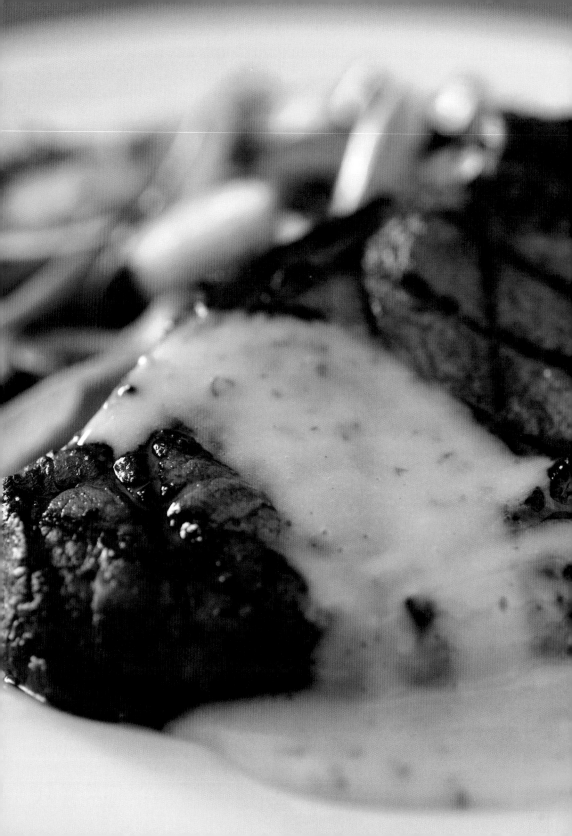

STEAK BÉARNAISE

A tasty entrée that never goes out of style.

MAKES 4 SERVINGS

4 (6-oz.) steaks, either filet mignon or cut of your choice
Salt and pepper
2 Tbsp. butter
1 Tbsp. olive oil

For Béarnaise Sauce:

2 Tbsp. mayonnaise
2 Tbsp. red wine vinegar
4 egg yolks
¼ cup fresh tarragon leaves, finely chopped
⅛ tsp. salt
2 sticks butter, cut into 2-Tbsp. pats

Preheat oven to 375° F.

Season both sides of the steaks generously with salt and pepper. In a large, heavy, ovenproof skillet, heat together the butter and olive oil over medium-high heat until butter has melted and foaming subsides. Place the steaks in the hot pan and cook until well seared on the first side, about 3 minutes. Turn the steaks and transfer the pan to the oven. Roast for about 5–8 minutes for medium rare. Remove from oven and let stand for 5 minutes, then place on serving plates.

Have ready a double boiler, or a pan of simmering water and a stainless steel or glass bowl that will act as a double boiler. Combine mayonnaise, vinegar, egg yolks, tarragon, and salt in the bowl of a blender or food processor.

Melt butter in a small saucepan until it begins to boil; do not let it start to brown. Turn on the blender or food processor and slowly pour in the melted butter.

Transfer sauce to the double boiler or bowl. Place over simmering water and stir constantly until sauce thickens, about 2 minutes.

Spoon béarnaise sauce over steaks and serve.

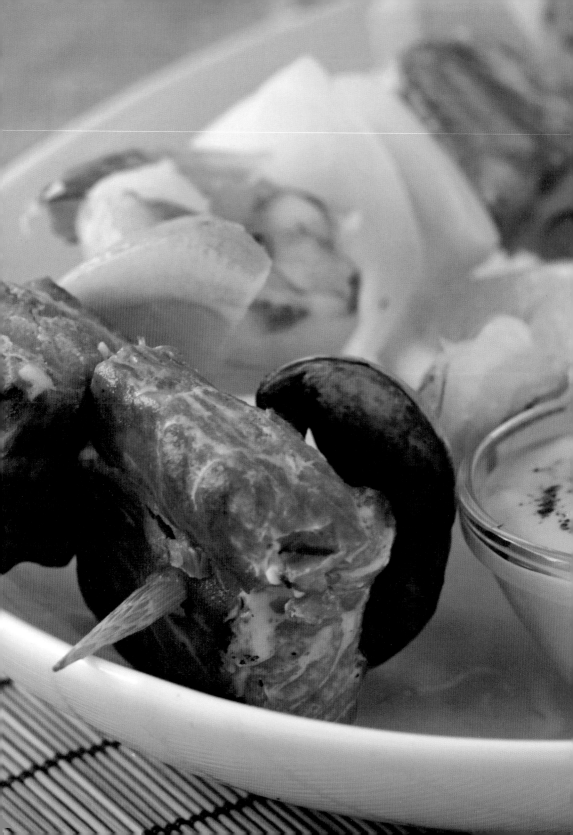

GRILLED SALMON AND SHRIMP KABOBS WITH CITRUS BBQ SAUCE

This is a great dish to make ahead for lunch, dinner, or a celebration.
Cook or grill when your guests arrive.

MAKES 4 SERVINGS

For Citrus BBQ Sauce:

1 cup prepared yellow mustard
2 Tbsp. balsamic vinegar
2 Tbsp. butter
1 Tbsp. Worcestershire sauce
2 Tbsp. lime juice
2 Tbsp. lemon juice
2 Tbsp. lemon zest
¼ tsp. cayenne pepper

For Salmon and Shrimp Kabobs:

8 jumbo shrimp, peeled and deveined
1 lb. center-cut salmon fillet
1 medium white or yellow onion
1 lemon
8 medium white mushrooms
Olive oil
Salt and pepper, to taste

If you would like the BBQ sauce a little sweeter, add 2 Tbsp. xylitol.

Combine Citrus BBQ Sauce ingredients in a medium saucepan. Bring to a boil over medium heat. Reduce heat and simmer for 20 minutes; set aside.

Cut salmon into 1" pieces the same thickness as the shrimp. Cut onion into 1" pieces. Cut lemon into 8 wedges the same thickness as the shrimp and salmon.

Preheat grill for direct cooking over medium heat. (Be sure to brush and oil the grate well before cooking.)

Alternate seafood and vegetables on bamboo skewers that have been soaking in water for at least 1 hour. Lightly brush with olive oil, then season with salt and pepper.

Cook on hot oiled grill for 2 minutes. Turn and brush with BBQ sauce. Cook an additional 2 minutes; turn and brush with more sauce. Repeat every minute until shrimp is opaque and salmon is cooked through. Total cooking time is 7–10 minutes.

Serve hot with additional BBQ sauce.

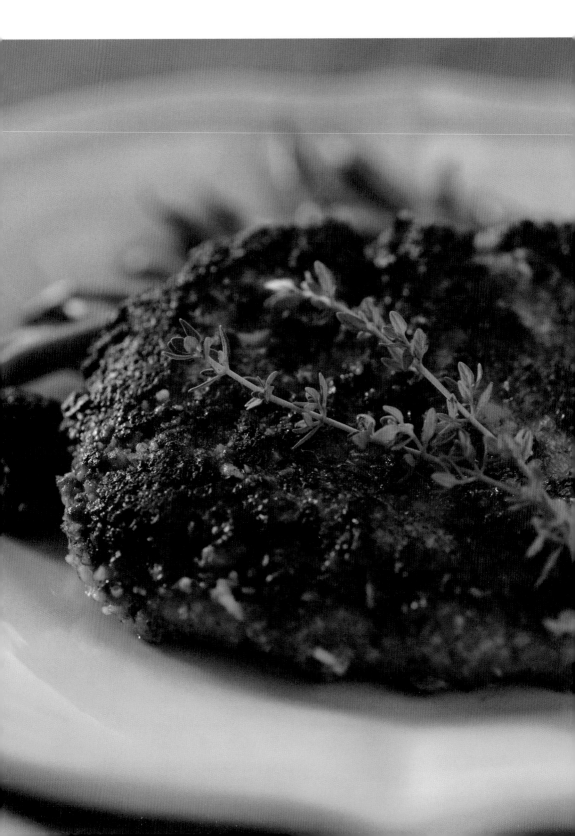

RASPBERRY DIJON PORK CHOPS

This coating also works on a firm fish fillet or boneless chicken breast.

MAKES 4 SERVINGS

4 center-cut pork loin chops
½ tsp. salt
¼ tsp. black pepper
¼ cup fresh or frozen raspberries
¼ cup Dijon mustard
½ cup very finely chopped walnuts (almost ground)
2 Tbsp. olive oil
¼ cup fresh raspberries, for garnish

If you would like this dish a little sweeter, add 2 Tbsp. xylitol.

With a meat mallet, pound pork chops between sheets of wax paper to ½" thickness. Season with salt and pepper.

Combine raspberries and mustard (and xylitol if desired) in a blender until smooth. Transfer to a shallow bowl.

Spread finely chopped walnuts on a plate. Coat pork chops with raspberry mustard, then roll each one in walnuts.

Heat oil in a large skillet over medium heat. Sauté pork chops until cooked through and crust is light brown, about 3–5 minutes on each side. Garnish with raspberries, and serve warm with your favorite green vegetable.

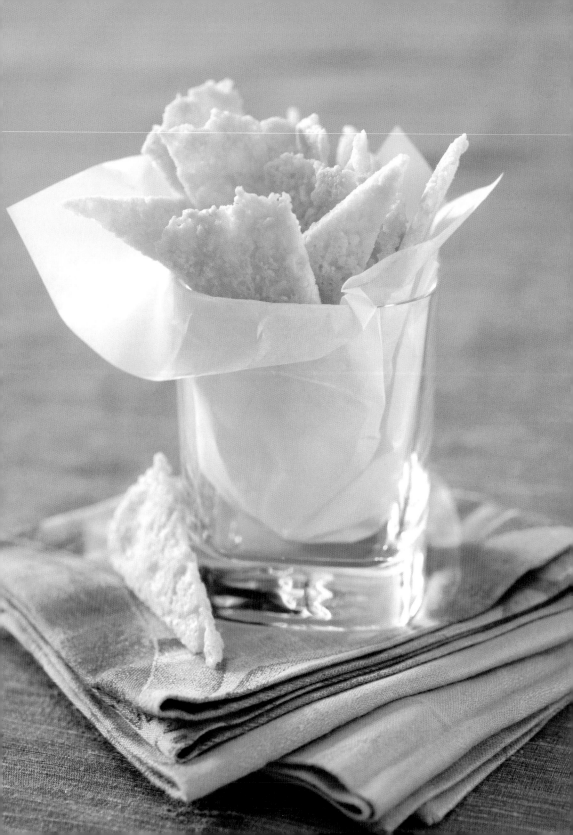

BELLY FAT CURE CHEESY PARMESAN CRISPS

The secret to these delicious and easy crisps is a nonstick or well-seasoned cast iron pan. These crisps are perfect served with dips, soups, or salads. Buy the pre-shredded Parmesan, not grated. The shredded Parmesan makes for a great crisp texture.

MAKES 4 SERVINGS

½ cup shredded Parmesan cheese

Heat an 8" pan over medium-low heat. Sprinkle cheese in an even layer, covering the bottom of the pan. Cook 2–3 minutes or until melted. Flip and cook 1 minute more. Remove cheese round from pan and place on a cutting board. While still warm, cut round in half with a sharp knife or pizza cutter. Cut each half into 6 wedges for a total of 12 crisps per round.

For croutons: Follow instructions above; while still warm, remove cheese from pan and roll into a log. Flatten the log with your hand, and cut into squares for croutons.

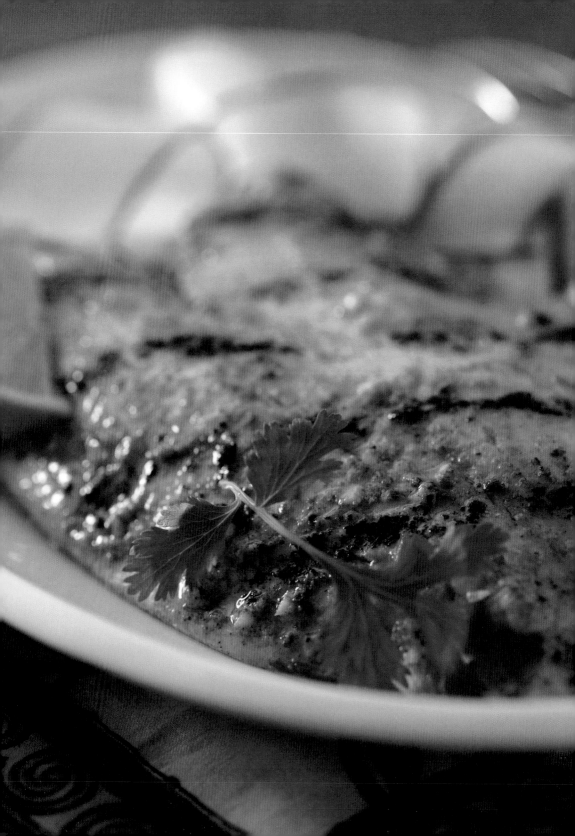

INDIAN SPICED GRILLED TILAPIA WITH ZUCCHINI RIBBONS

Beautiful colors and flavors make this dish an international favorite.

MAKES 4 SERVINGS

4 tilapia fillets
¼ cup olive oil
2 Tbsp. lemon juice
4 cloves garlic, minced
1 Tbsp. minced fresh ginger
1 tsp. ground turmeric
1 tsp. ground cumin
1 tsp. dried thyme
¼ tsp. cayenne pepper
Pinch ground cloves

Pinch ground cinnamon
½ tsp. black pepper
½ tsp. salt
¼ cup plain Greek yogurt
2 Tbsp. chopped cilantro, for garnish

For Ribbons:

2 medium zucchini
2 Tbsp. butter

Place tilapia fillets in a large zip-top bag. Stir together remaining ingredients, except cilantro, in a medium bowl and pour into bag with fish. Gently massage bag to coat fish with marinade, then seal bag. Marinate in refrigerator for 30 minutes or up to 4 hours.

Remove fish from refrigerator about 30 minutes before cooking. Remove fillets from marinade and shake off any excess. Discard marinade.

While fillets come to room temperature, cut off ends of zucchini. Use a vegetable peeler down the length of each zucchini to make "ribbons."

Preheat grill for direct cooking over medium heat. (Be sure to brush and oil the grate well before cooking.)

Cook fish for 5 minutes per side or until it is cooked through and flakes easily with a fork. Transfer to serving platter and cover loosely with foil.

Melt butter in a medium skillet. Sauté zucchini ribbons for 2–3 minutes.

Serve grilled tilapia and zucchini immediately. Garnish with cilantro.

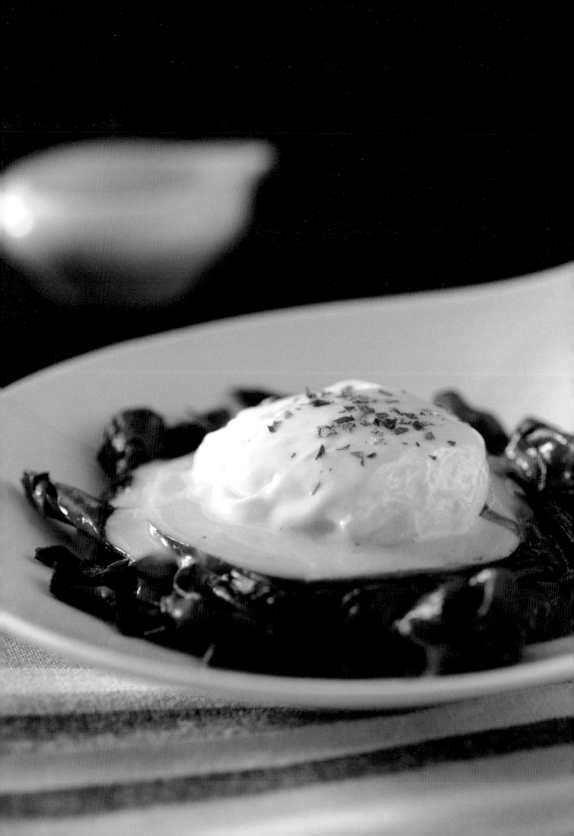

FARM EGGS BENEDICT

You can substitute sautéed spinach or kale for the red chard.

MAKES 4 SERVINGS

For Hollandaise Sauce:

2 Tbsp. mayonnaise
2 Tbsp. lemon juice
4 egg yolks
⅛ tsp. salt
1 pinch cayenne powder
2 sticks butter, cut into 2-Tbsp. pats

Have ready:

4 slices Canadian bacon
4 large eggs, poached*
1 bunch red chard, sautéed**

Have ready a double boiler, or a pan of simmering water and a stainless steel or glass bowl that will act as a double boiler. Combine mayonnaise, lemon juice, egg yolks, salt, and cayenne pepper in the bowl of a blender or food processor. Melt butter in a small saucepan until it begins to boil; do not let it start to brown. Turn on the blender or food processor and slowly pour in the melted butter. Transfer to your bowl for the double boiler. Place over simmering water and stir constantly until sauce thickens, about 2 minutes.

To serve, stack warmed Canadian bacon and a poached egg on top of sautéed red chard. Top with hollandaise sauce and a sprinkle of cayenne pepper, if desired.

*To poach an egg, bring 1½" of water to a boil in a skillet. Reduce the heat so that the water is barely simmering (bubbles not breaking the surface). Crack an egg into a small bowl and, placing the lip of the bowl at the surface of the water, slide the egg into the water. Repeat with remaining eggs; work in two batches if necessary. Poach eggs for 3–5 minutes or until the whites are firm.

**Rinse and dry 1 bunch red chard. Remove stems and cut into 2" pieces; roughly chop leaves. Heat 1½ Tbsp. olive oil in a large skillet. Add stem and sauté for about 5 minutes or until fork tender. Add leaves and sauté until wilted.

Season with salt and pepper.

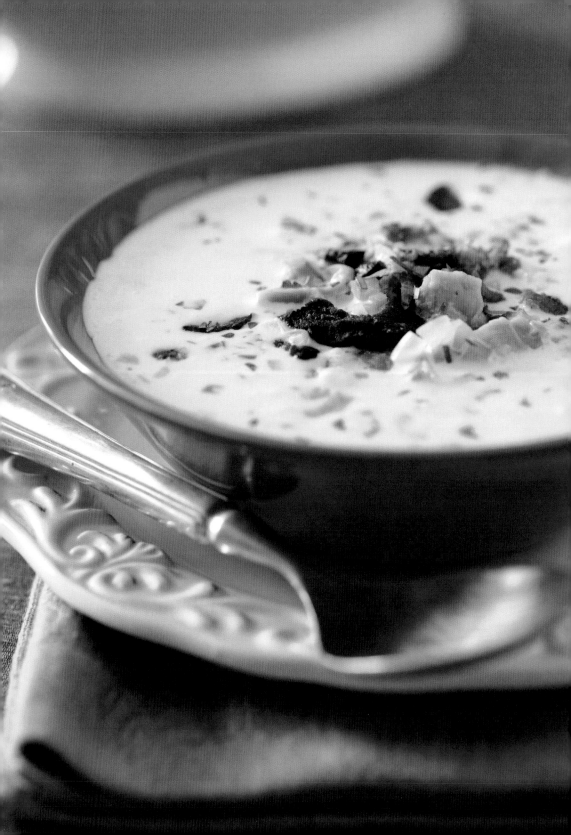

NEW ENGLAND–STYLE CLAM CHOWDER

Celery root takes the place of potatoes in this white and creamy-style chowder.

MAKES 4 GENEROUS SERVINGS

3 slices thick-cut bacon, chopped
1 medium onion, finely chopped
2 celery ribs, finely chopped
2 cloves garlic, minced
3 cups chicken stock
2 cups diced celery root
½ tsp. salt
3 cups half-and-half
4 (6½-oz.) cans chopped clams, with their juices
2 Tbsp. fresh parsley, finely chopped
3 Tbsp. butter
Salt and pepper, to taste

Cook bacon in a large pot over medium heat until browned, but not crispy. Remove bacon with a slotted spoon and set aside. Add onion, celery ribs, and garlic; sauté until vegetables are soft. Stir in stock, celery root, and salt. Cover and cook chowder until celery root is cooked but still firm. (Test by poking with a fork.)

Add half-and-half, reserved bacon, clams (including juices), parsley, and butter; simmer for 3 minutes more.

Season to taste with salt and pepper. Serve hot.

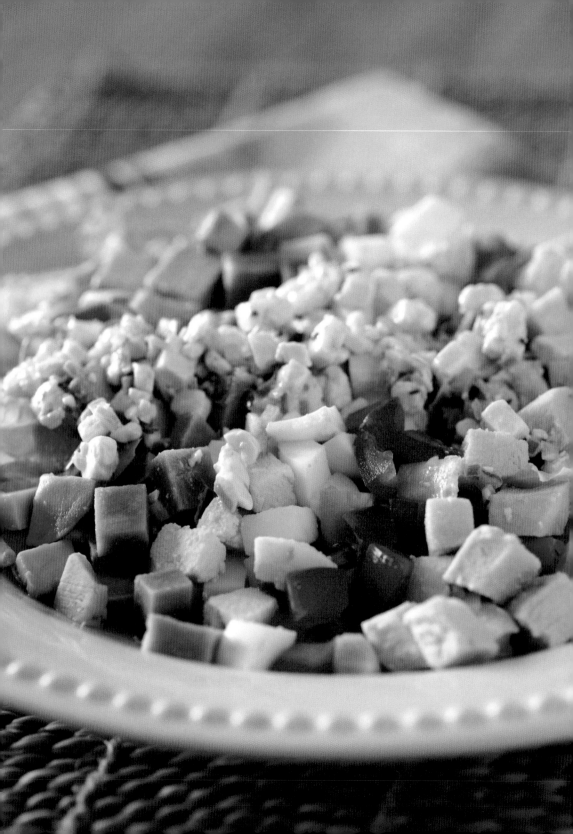

BELLY FAT CURE CHOPPED SALAD

A classic recipe perfect for lunch or Sunday brunch.

MAKES 4 SERVINGS

For Dressing:

2 Tbsp. chopped shallots
½ tsp. dried oregano
½ tsp. dried basil
2 Tbsp. red wine vinegar
3–4 dashes hot sauce
⅓ cup olive oil
½ cup good-quality blue cheese
Salt and pepper, to taste

For Salad:

1 head romaine lettuce, chopped into ¼"-wide strips
4 hard-boiled eggs, chopped
2 avocados, diced
1 Roma tomato, seeded and diced
2 green onions, sliced
1½ cups diced turkey breast
1½ cups diced ham

For dressing, combine shallots, dried oregano, dried basil, red wine vinegar, and hot sauce in a small bowl. Slowly whisk in olive oil until combined. Crumble blue cheese and stir in; season with salt and pepper to taste. Chill for an hour.

Arrange the salad ingredients on chilled plates. Spoon dressing over salads and serve.

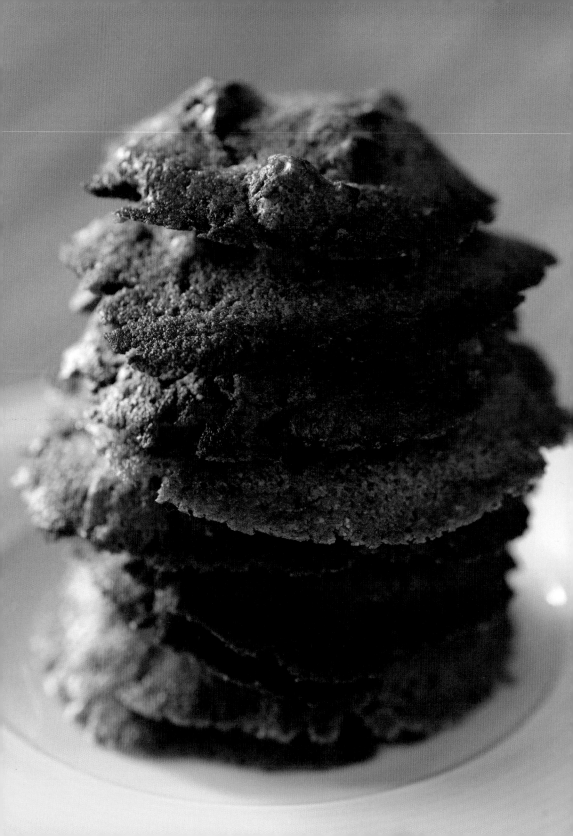

JORGE'S CHOCOLATE LACE COOKIES

These delicate cookies' edges look like lace.

MAKES 24 COOKIES

2 sticks butter, softened
⅔ cup xylitol
1 tsp. vanilla extract
2 large eggs
1 cup almond flour (about ½ cup almonds ground in a coffee grinder)
¼ cup unsweetened cocoa powder
1 cup stevia-sweetened whey protein powder
1 tsp. baking powder
½ tsp. salt
4 oz. dark chocolate (85% or greater), chopped
1 cup chopped walnuts

Preheat oven to 350° F. Line a baking sheet with parchment paper; set aside.

Beat together butter, xylitol, and vanilla extract until light and fluffy. Beat in eggs one at a time.

Whisk together almond flour, cocoa powder, whey powder, baking powder, and salt in a separate bowl. Stir dry ingredients into butter mixture. Stir in chopped walnuts and chocolate until combined.

Spoon heaping teaspoons of batter 2" apart on prepared baking sheet. Place in freezer for 5 minutes. Remove and bake for 9–10 minutes. Cookies will be lacy and spread during baking. Cool cookies completely on baking sheet.

Store in an airtight container—these cookies crumble when exposed to air.

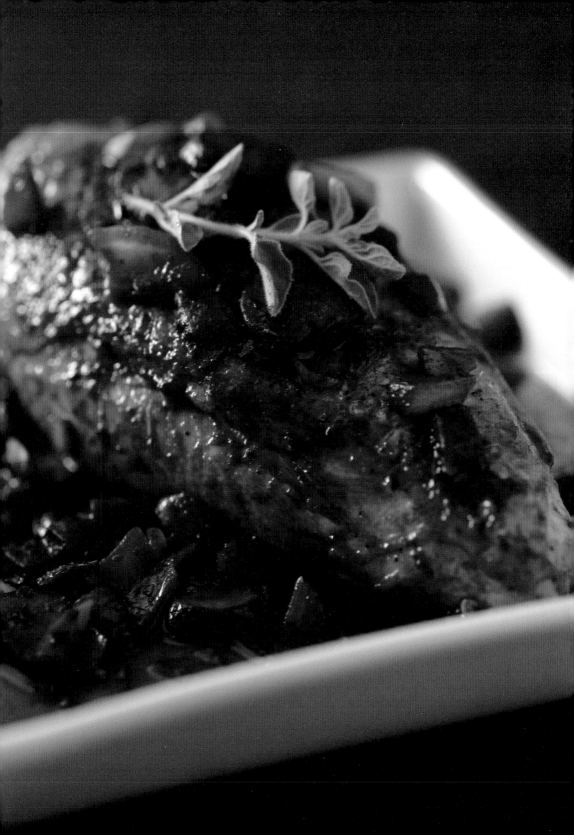

CHICKEN CACCIATORE

This is a great-tasting and comforting recipe, perfect for a Sunday-night dinner.

MAKES 4 SERVINGS

3 Tbsp. olive oil
4 bone-in chicken breasts with skin
Salt and pepper, to taste
1 medium onion, chopped
12 oz. cremini mushrooms, sliced
2 garlic cloves, chopped
1 bay leaf
½ tsp. dried oregano
½ tsp. dried basil
¼ tsp. dried thyme
½ tsp. crushed red pepper
¾ cup red wine
1½ cup chicken broth
2 Tbsp. organic tomato paste

Heat oil in a large skillet over medium-high heat. Season chicken breasts with salt and pepper and cook, skin-side down, until golden brown. Remove and set aside. Reduce heat to medium and sauté onion, mushrooms, and garlic in the same skillet. Stir in remaining ingredients and bring to a boil. Return chicken to skillet, cover, and reduce heat to low. Simmer for 35 minutes.

Remove chicken breasts. Bring sauce to a boil and reduce by half. Return chicken to the pan and coat with sauce. Serve with remaining sauce.

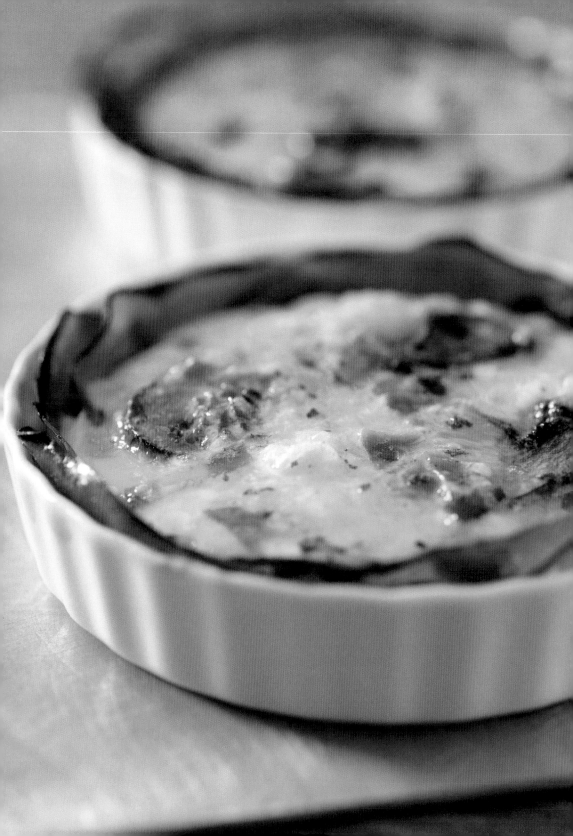

HAM-CRUSTED BREAKFAST QUICHE

For a fun presentation, make this quiche in single-serving quiche pans.

MAKES 6 SERVINGS

6 oz. smoked ham, thinly sliced
1 cup half-and-half
6 eggs
Salt and pepper, to taste
Pinch nutmeg (optional)
½ cup mushrooms, sliced
1 small leek—white part only, finely chopped
1 cup Swiss cheese, grated

Preheat oven to 425° F.

Line a 9" pie dish with overlapping slices of ham. Cut off any excess ham that hangs over. Chop the excess ham and set aside.

In a medium bowl, combine eggs, half-and-half, salt, and pepper (and nutmeg if you choose) until well mixed but not foamy. Add mushrooms, leek, Swiss cheese, and any reserved chopped ham. Pour slowly into ham-lined pie plate.

Bake at 425° F for 15 minutes, then reduce heat to 325° and bake until a knife inserted into the center comes out clean, about 25–30 minutes.

Serve warm.

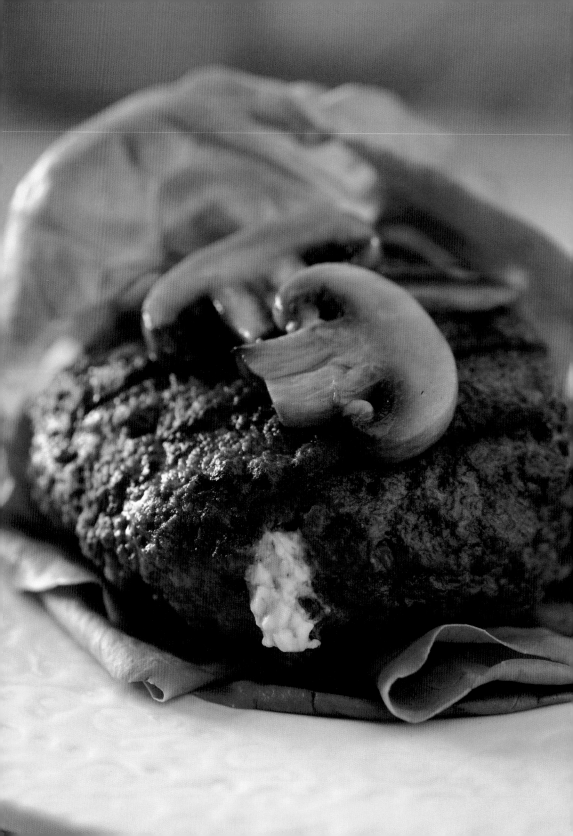

BLACK AND BLUE BURGERS

Limestone or butter lettuce also makes a great "hamburger roll."

MAKES 4 SERVINGS

4 oz. good-quality blue cheese (not the precrumbled kind)
4 oz. butter, softened
1½ lbs. ground chuck
Blackened seasoning
Olive oil
Salt and pepper, to taste
1 Tbsp. butter
4 oz. mushrooms
4 outer leaves butter lettuce
Dijon mustard, for serving

Crumble blue cheese into a bowl. Add 4 oz. butter and mash together with a fork. Place mixture on a piece of plastic wrap and shape into a 2"-diameter log. Wrap in plastic and refrigerate until firm.

Divide ground beef into 8 equal patties. Slice the blue cheese butter into thin pieces and place on 4 of the burger patties, leaving a border. Top each burger with another patty. Pinch the edges together firmly and reshape into a round patty of even thickness. Generously season both sides and edges of the burgers with blackened seasoning. Cover and refrigerate until ready to cook.

Preheat grill for direct cooking over high heat. (Be sure to brush and oil the grate well before cooking.)

While the grill is heating, heat a medium skillet over medium-high heat and add 1 Tbsp. butter. When the butter is melted and foaming subsides, add mushrooms; salt and pepper to taste. Turn the heat down to medium and continue to cook for about 6–7 minutes or until the mushrooms are nicely browned.

While the mushrooms are cooking, place the burgers on the grill and cook for about 5 minutes per side, or until the center of the meat registers 160° F with a meat thermometer.

Serve burgers wrapped in lettuce leaves and topped with Dijon mustard and sautéed mushrooms.

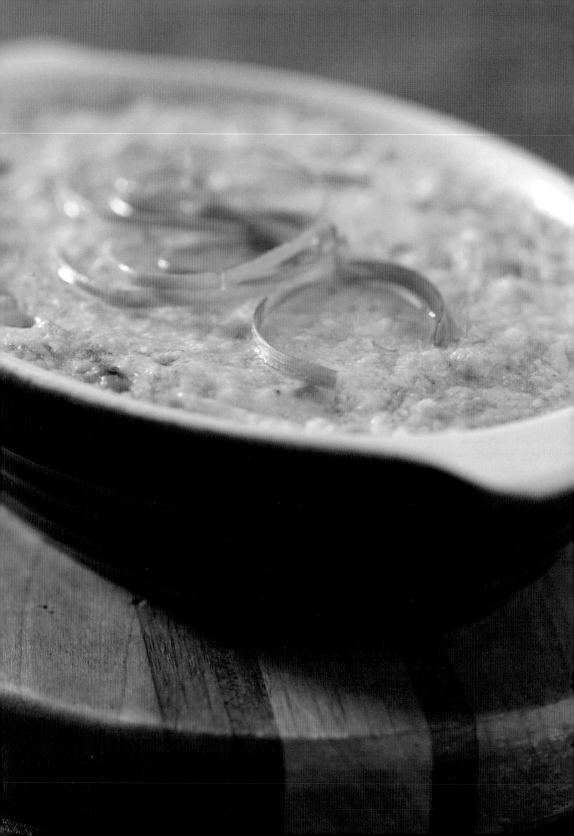

BAKED ARTICHOKE DIP

This delicious dip is perfect for serving with raw vegetables or Parmesan Crisps.

MAKES 4 SERVINGS

2 (14-oz.) cans artichoke hearts, drained and chopped
4 green onions, chopped
3 cloves garlic, chopped
½ cup mayonnaise
½ cup sour cream
½ cup grated Parmesan cheese
2 Tbsp. lemon juice
¼ tsp. cayenne pepper
⅓ cup olive oil
Salt and pepper, to taste

Preheat oven to 350° F. Spray a 1-quart baking dish with olive oil cooking spray; set aside.

Place all chopped artichokes, green onions, and garlic in a food processor and pulse until finely chopped. Add mayonnaise, sour cream, Parmesan cheese, lemon juice, and cayenne pepper; pulse until just combined. With motor running, slowly pour in olive oil until thoroughly blended.

Season to taste with salt and pepper; transfer to prepared baking dish. Bake in preheated oven 40–45 minutes, until the mixture is set and top is golden brown.

Serve warm.

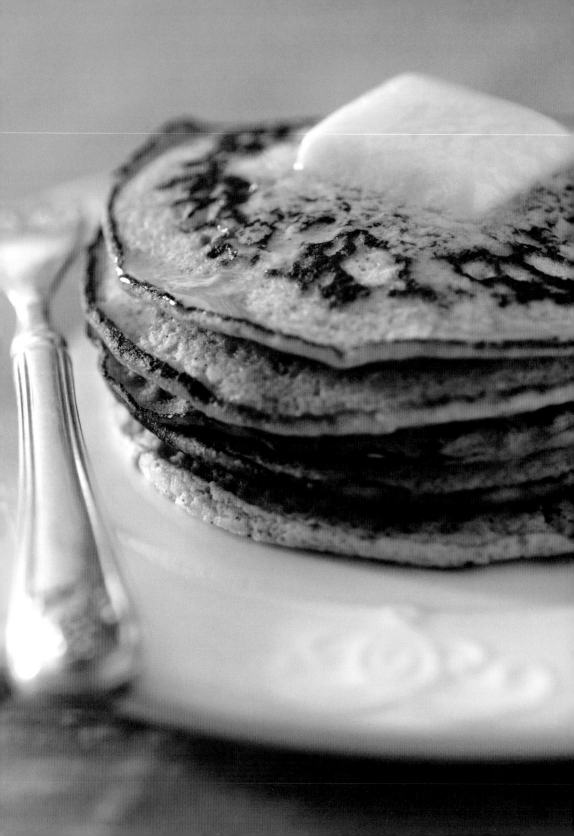

SWEET RICOTTA PANCAKES

Delicious breakfast pancakes without any flour.

MAKES 4 SERVINGS

2½ cups ricotta cheese
8 large eggs
2 tsp. vanilla extract
⅓ cup xylitol
2 tsp. cinnamon
¾ tsp. salt
1½ Tbsp. coconut oil
Butter, for garnish
Fresh raspberries, for garnish

Place ricotta in a medium mixing bowl and beat in the eggs, one at a time, with a wooden spoon. Stir in vanilla extract, xylitol, cinnamon, and salt.

Heat the oil in a large skillet over medium heat. Working in batches, ladle the batter to make 6 pancakes. Cook until the pancakes set, about 4 or 5 minutes. (Note that the surface of the pancakes will still be a little soft.) Flip pancakes and finish cooking, about 1–2 minutes more.

Can be kept warm in 200° F oven until ready to serve with butter and berries.

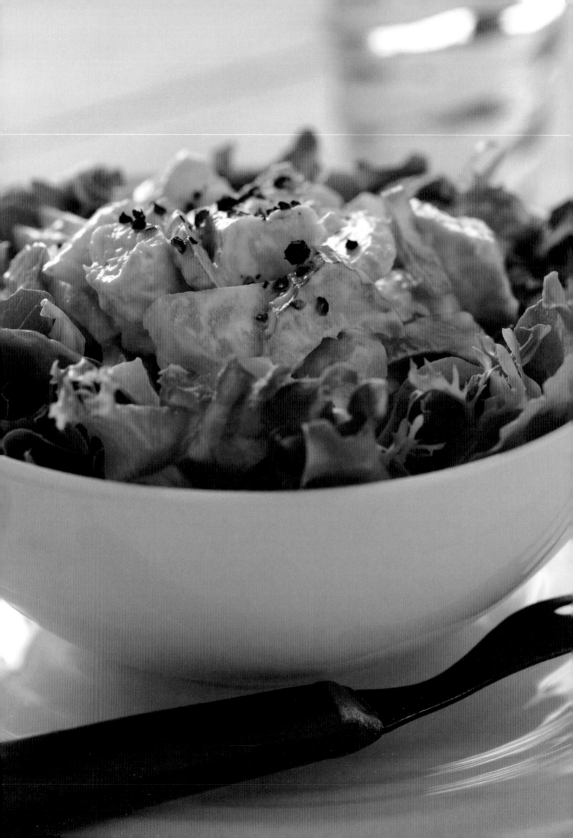

AMAZING ASIAN SALAD

Water chestnuts add a delicious crunch to this tasty salad.

MAKES 4 SERVINGS

2 cups cooked chicken, diced
1 cup chopped celery
1 (16-oz.) can water chestnuts, drained and chopped
⅓ cup mayonnaise
1 Tbsp. soy sauce
1 tsp. lemon juice
8 cups mixed greens

In a large bowl, combine the chicken, celery, and water chestnuts.

In a separate bowl, combine the mayonnaise, soy sauce, and lemon juice.

Add the dressing to the chicken mixture and toss. Cover and refrigerate if desired.

For each serving, place a scoop of the chicken salad onto a 2-cup bed of mixed greens.

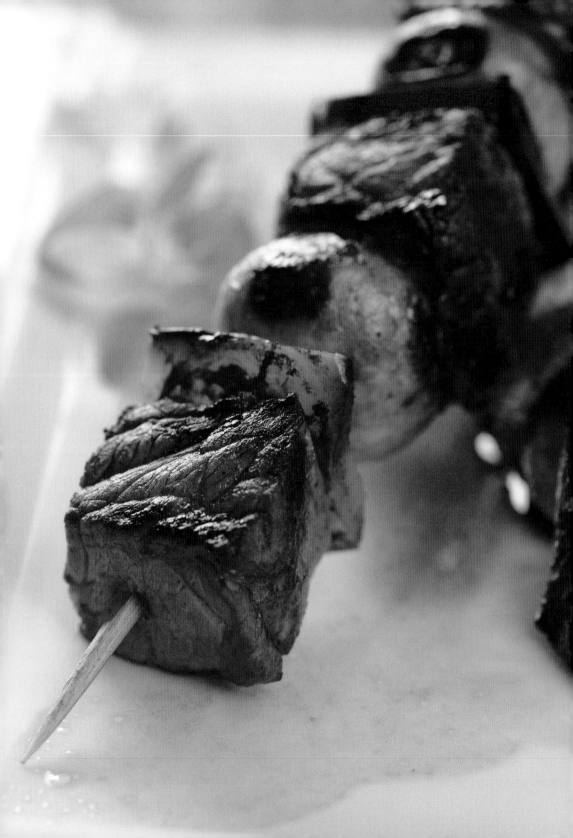

BEEFY KABOBS

These grilled beef kabobs are sure to satisfy.

MAKES 4 SERVINGS

2 tsp. olive oil
¼ cup red wine vinegar
1 Tbsp. soy sauce
1 garlic clove, minced
1½ lbs. top sirloin steak, cut into 24 cubes
1 medium red bell pepper, cut into 1" pieces
1 medium yellow bell pepper, cut into 1" pieces
½ lb. mushrooms, stems removed

Combine the first four ingredients in a bowl. Add beef cubes and marinate in the refrigerator for at least 3 hours.

Soak 8 wooden skewers in water briefly. Thread beef cubes, mushroom caps, and pepper slices on each skewer. Baste with marinade and transfer to grill; cook over medium heat.

Halfway through cooking, turn and baste each skewer with marinade; continue grilling until done. Transfer to plate.

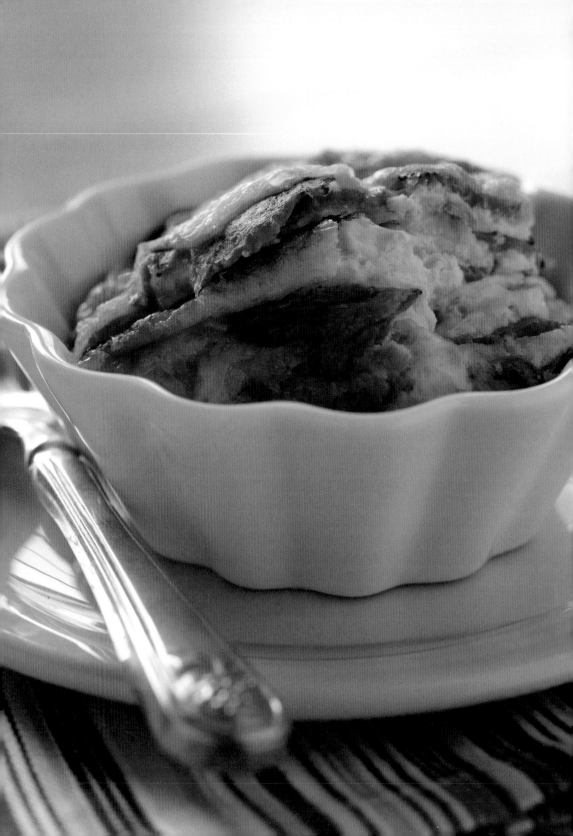

BRUNCH TIME CHILI BAKE

Excellent with a salad of mixed greens with olive oil-and-vinegar dressing.

MAKES 4 SERVINGS

1 (27-oz.) can whole green chilies, drained
¾ cup shredded cheddar cheese
¾ cup shredded Jack cheese
5 eggs, lightly beaten
¼ cup heavy cream
Salt and pepper, to taste

Preheat oven to 350° F. Grease an 8" x 12" baking dish.

Slice chili peppers open and remove all seeds; pat dry.

Line the bottom of the dish with one layer of green chilies topped with some shredded cheese. Repeat layering process.

In medium bowl, whisk together eggs and heavy cream. Season with salt and pepper and pour evenly over chilies and cheese.

Bake for 30 minutes, or until filling is set. Let stand for 10 minutes before serving.

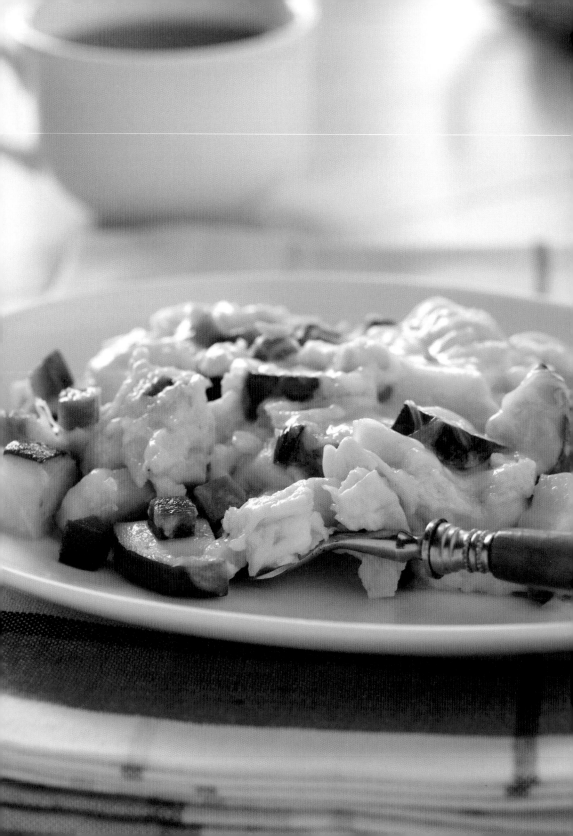

HAM AND SWISS SCRAMBLE

A robust mix of flavors makes this a scrumptious breakfast.

MAKES 4 SERVINGS

4 Tbsp. butter
1 cup zucchini, chopped
1 cup red bell pepper, chopped
8 eggs
¼ cup heavy cream
Salt and pepper, to taste
1 cup ham, diced
1 cup Swiss cheese, shredded

Melt butter in a large skillet over medium heat. Add zucchini and bell pepper. Cook until tender. Remove from skillet and set aside.

Whisk eggs together with cream, salt, and pepper. Add the egg mixture to the skillet and scramble until eggs are cooked almost through.

Add the vegetable mixture, diced ham, and cheese to the skillet and continue scrambling until eggs are cooked through.

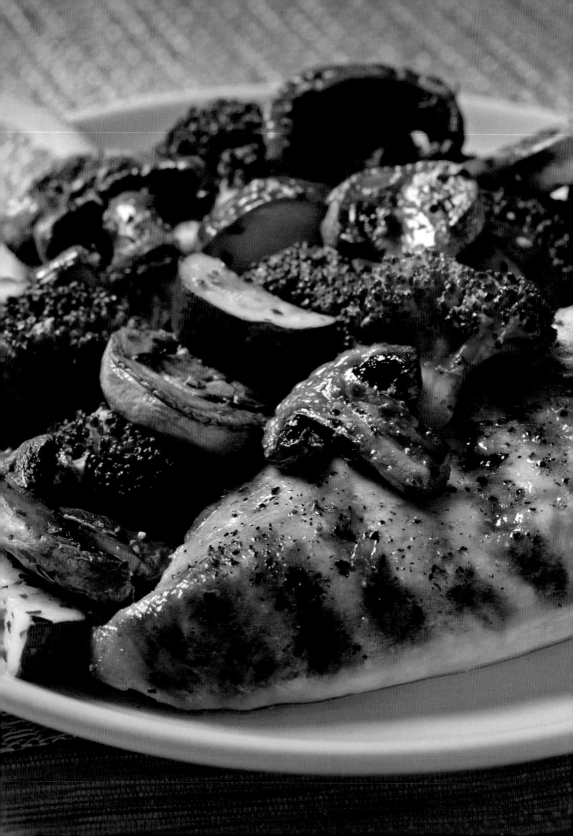

LEMON CHICKEN WITH ROASTED VEGETABLES

The lemon flavor of this chicken pairs nicely with roasted Italian vegetables.

MAKES 4 SERVINGS

3 Tbsp. lemon juice
5 Tbsp. olive oil
1 Tbsp. Italian seasoning
Salt and pepper, to taste
1½ cups zucchini, cut into 1" chunks
1½ cups broccoli florets
½ lb. button mushrooms, halved
4 chicken breasts, boneless and skinless

Preheat oven to 400° F. Grease an 8" x 12" baking dish. Place chicken in baking dish.

Mix lemon juice and 2 Tbsp. olive oil in a small bowl. Brush the tops of the chicken breasts with oil mixture.

Combine remaining oil and seasonings in a small bowl. Place vegetables in baking dish and drizzle oil mixture over vegetables.

Bake for 40–45 minutes, turning vegetables occasionally.

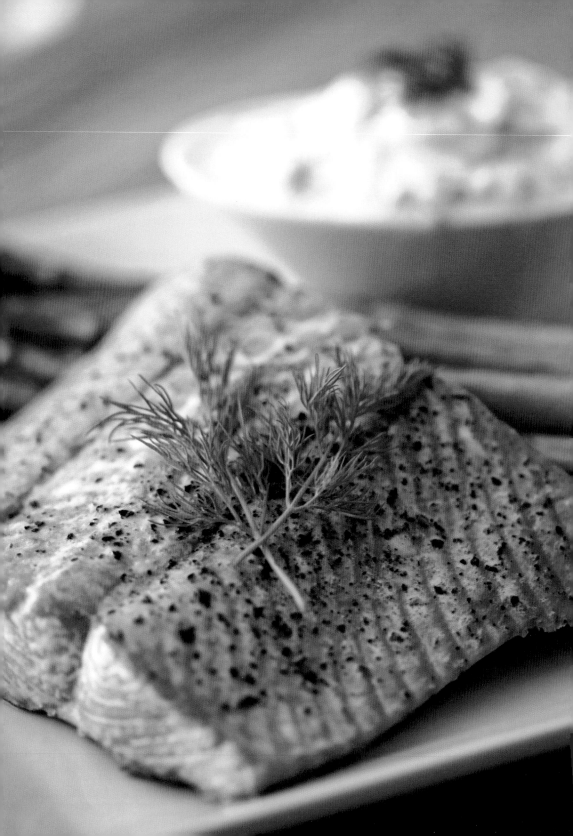

SALMON WITH DILL SAUCE AND ASPARAGUS

A delicious meal with exceptional nutritional value.

MAKES 4 SERVINGS

1 lb. asparagus, ends trimmed
3 Tbsp. olive oil
Salt and pepper, to taste
4 salmon fillets, 5 oz. each
1 tsp. balsamic vinegar

For Dill Sauce:

½ cup Greek yogurt
2 Tbsp. mayonnaise
1 garlic clove, minced
2 Tbsp. heavy cream
1 tsp. chopped fresh dill
¼ tsp. dried oregano

Preheat oven to 425° F. Cover a baking sheet with foil. Toss asparagus with 2 Tbsp. olive oil and place to one side of baking sheet.

Rub each salmon fillet all over with remaining 1 Tbsp. olive oil, season with salt and pepper, and place on other side of baking sheet.

Roast salmon and asparagus for 13–15 minutes or until fish is just cooked through.

Combine yogurt, mayonnaise, garlic, heavy cream, dill, and oregano in a small bowl and chill in refrigerator.

Place a quarter of the asparagus on each serving plate and drizzle with balsamic vinegar. Place 1 salmon fillet on each plate beside the asparagus and serve with 1 Tbsp. chilled dill sauce.

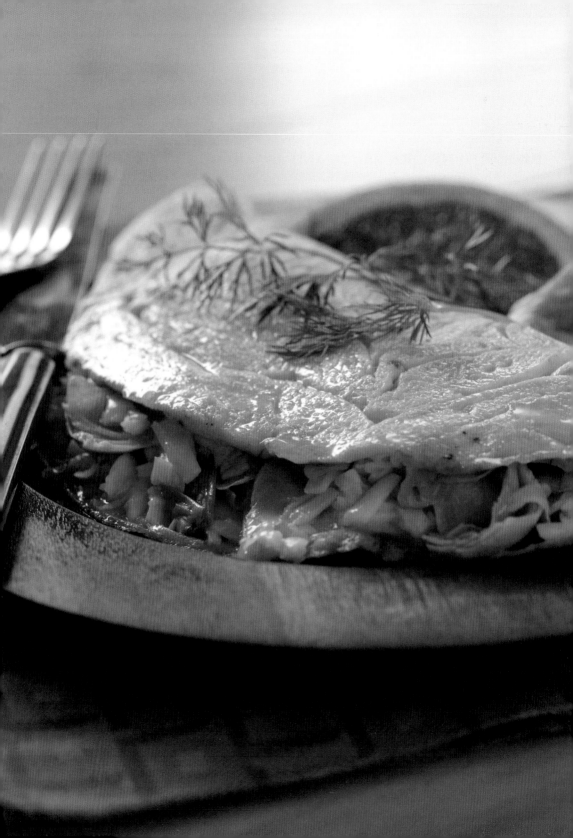

SMOKY GOUDA OMELETTE

Artichoke hearts and smoked Gouda cheese make an interesting combination.

MAKES 4 SERVINGS

8 eggs
Salt and pepper, to taste
¼ cup butter, divided
½ cup marinated artichoke hearts, drained and chopped
¾ cup smoked Gouda cheese, shredded

Whisk eggs together with salt and pepper.

Melt butter in a small skillet over medium heat. Add a quarter of the egg mixture and cook until the eggs begin to set on the bottom of the pan. Gently lift the edges of the omelette with a spatula to allow any unset egg to flow to the edges and cook.

Top the eggs with a quarter of the artichoke hearts and Gouda cheese. Using a spatula, gently fold one side of the omelette over the other. Continue cooking until the cheese is melted.

Slide the omelette out of the skillet onto a plate. Repeat with remaining ingredients.

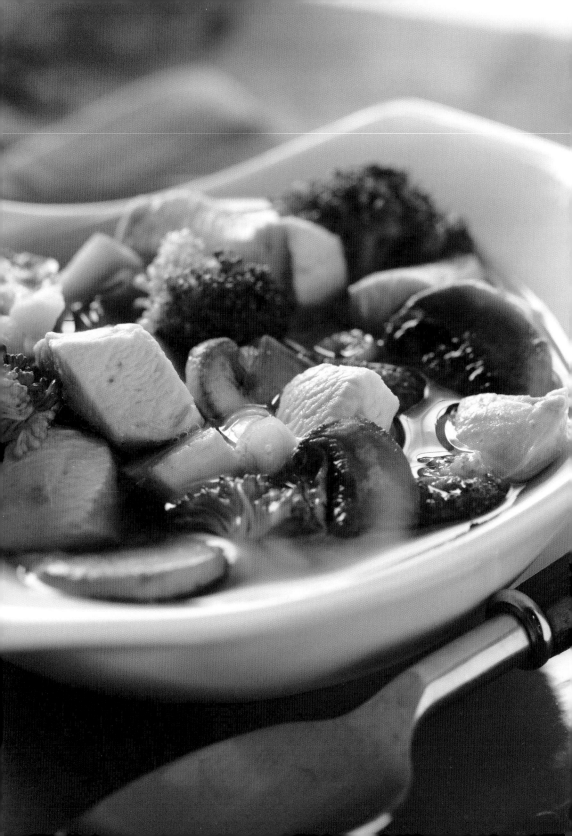

CHICKEN AND VEGGIE SOUP

Serve this hearty soup alongside a salad with olive oil-and-vinegar dressing

MAKES 4 SERVINGS

1 qt. chicken broth
1 Tbsp. soy sauce
1 cup sliced mushrooms
1 cup broccoli florets, chopped
2 Tbsp. green onions, finely chopped
2 precooked chicken breasts, cubed

Simmer first 5 ingredients in a large pot for 8 minutes.

Add cubed chicken and simmer an additional 8 minutes.

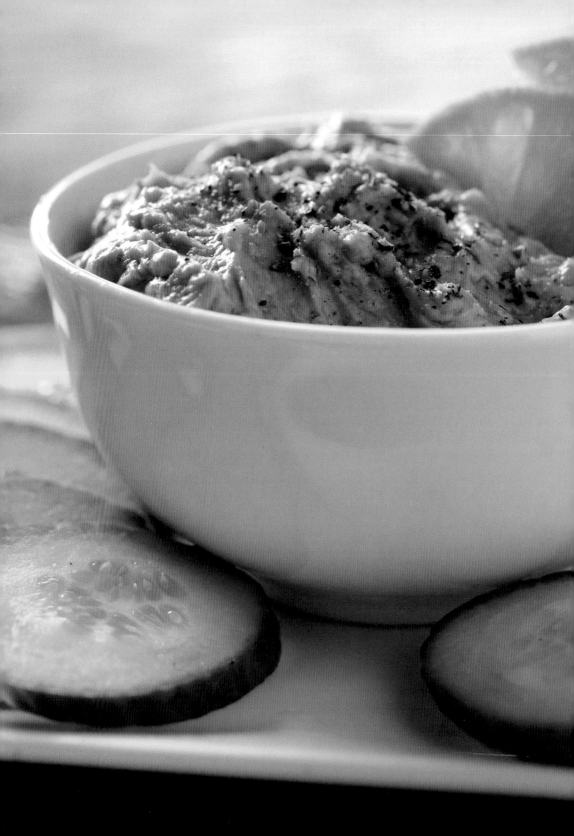

CHRISTY'S CREAMY GUACAMOLE

All the flavor and crunch you need.

MAKES 4 SERVINGS

4 large avocados
2 Tbsp. lime juice
1 jalapeño, diced (optional)
½ cup sour cream
Salt and pepper, to taste
1 large cucumber

Add the avocados, lime juice, sour cream, salt, and pepper (and jalapeño, if you wish) to bowl; mix and mash thoroughly.

Cut cucumber horizontally into slices that are about ⅛" thick. Dip the cucumber chips in the guacamole for a flavorful crunch.

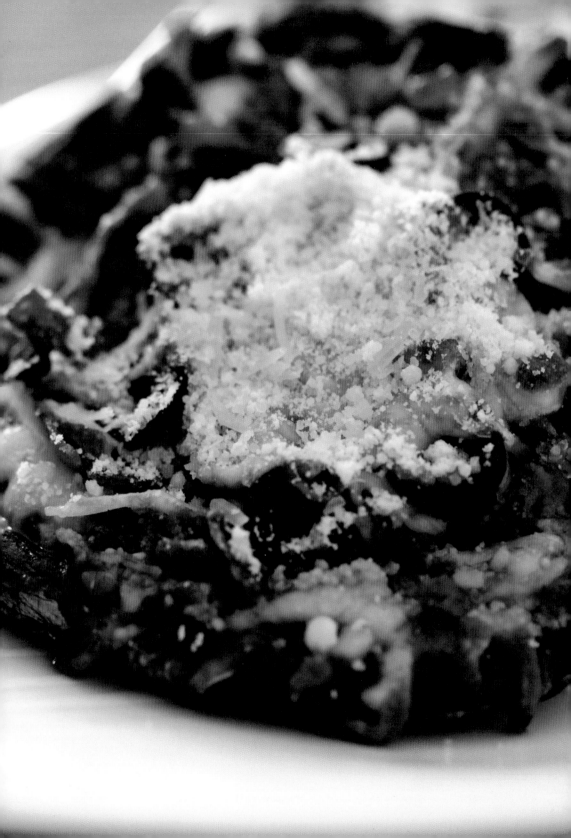

RYAN'S PORTOBELLO MINI-PIZZAS

This creative dish is easy and impressive.

MAKES 4 SERVINGS

8 large portobello mushrooms
8 Tbsp. pesto sauce (2 grams of sugar per serving or less)
Mozzarella cheese, shredded
12 black olives, sliced
8 strips of bacon, chopped
Parmesan cheese

Preheat oven to 450° F.

Grill portobello mushrooms on both sides. Allow them to cool and drain. Pat them dry and scrape out the black fins to create your mini pizza "crusts."

Cook the bacon to desired crispiness, then chop into small pieces.

Spread 1 Tbsp. of pesto sauce on the inside of each mushroom.

Top each mushroom with a layer of mozzarella cheese; add the sliced black olives and chopped bacon on top.

Finally, top each mushroom with Parmesan cheese and bake for 5 minutes, or until cheese is melted.

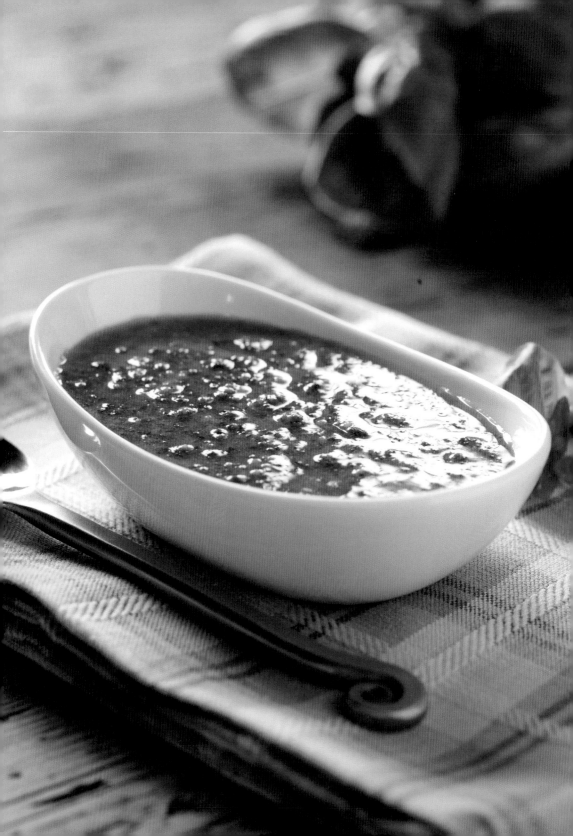

FRESH PESTO SAUCE

Defeat hidden sugar found in packaged pesto by quickly making yours from scratch.

MAKES 2 CUPS

3 cups fresh basil leaves
1½ cups walnuts, chopped
4 cloves garlic, peeled
1 cup olive oil
Salt and pepper, to taste

In a food processor, blend together the basil leaves, nuts, and garlic. Pour oil in slowly while continuing to mix.

Stir in salt and pepper to taste.

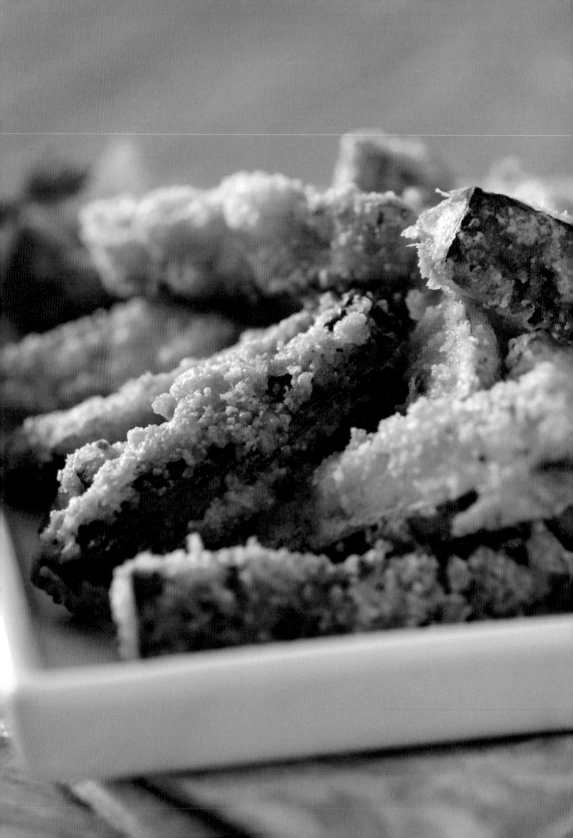

ZUCCHINI CHEESE FRIES

A much tastier and far healthier alternative to French fries.

MAKES 6–8 SERVINGS

8–10 medium zucchini
4 large eggs
1 Tbsp. chili powder
2 cups grated Parmesan cheese
Oil for frying

Preheat oven to 200° F.

Trim ends off zucchini, and cut each in half. Cut each zucchini half lengthwise into 3 wedges. Set aside. Combine eggs and chili powder in a shallow bowl and beat together. Spread grated Parmesan cheese on a plate.

Heat 1" oil in a large skillet, to 375° F. Dip zucchini fries into the egg mixture, and then coat with Parmesan cheese. Cook in preheated oil, in small batches, until golden brown. Keep in warm oven until ready to serve.

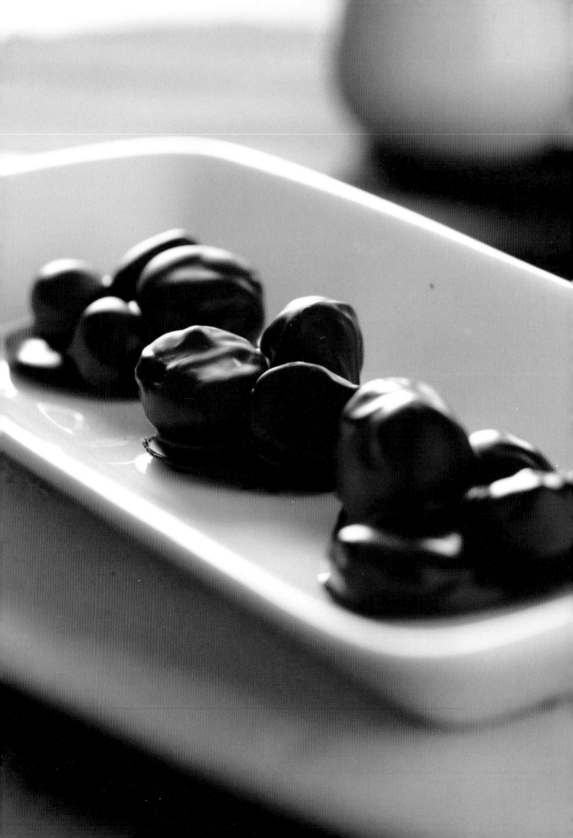

MACADAMIA NUT CLUSTERS

So rich that one is enough . . .

MAKES 12 CLUSTERS

3 oz. (approx. half of a large-size bar) dark chocolate (85% or greater)
1 tsp. butter
1 cup macadamia nuts
Salt (optional)

Microwave chocolate and butter in a medium-size glass bowl for 1 minute, stirring every 15 seconds (or use double boiler). Add 1 cup of macadamia nuts to chocolate mixture and stir to cover.

Drop mixture by rounded teaspoons onto tray covered with wax paper. Salt lightly if desired.

Refrigerate for 45 minutes, and enjoy.

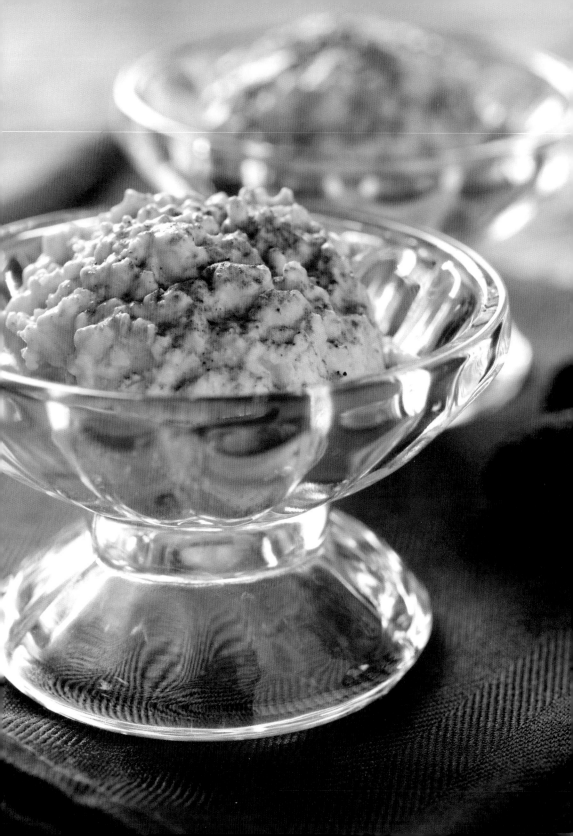

SWEET SURPRISE COTTAGE CHEESE

This cool, sweet treat is perfect for warmer months.

MAKES 4 SERVINGS

2 cups cottage cheese (not fat-free or low-fat)
1 Tbsp. plus 1 tsp. unsweetened cocoa powder, divided
2 packets xylitol, erythritol, or plain stevia

Place cottage cheese in a medium mixing bowl. Add 1 Tbsp. of cocoa powder and the 2 packets of sweetener. Mix well.

Divide cottage cheese mixture among 4 serving bowls and sprinkle with remaining cocoa powder.

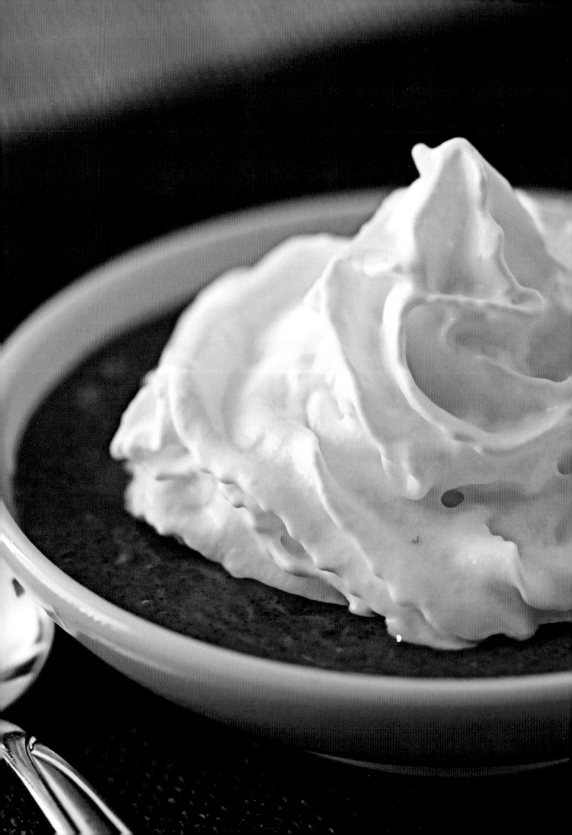

ITTY BITTY NUTTY PIE

This speedy sweet treat tastes like a Thanksgiving dessert.

MAKES 4 SERVINGS

4 heaping Tbsp. almond butter (creamy or chunky)
Low-sugar whipped cream
4 very small plates

Put one heaping scoop of almond butter on each small plate. Smooth the almond butter over the plate, leaving at least ½" between the almond butter and edge of the plate.

Cover the almond butter with a moderate amount of whipped cream . . . a 3-second squirt will do.

A little extra whipped cream at the center will hold a candle for special occasions, and with some creativity and variation in size, this toss-together favorite becomes a fun template for customized treats.

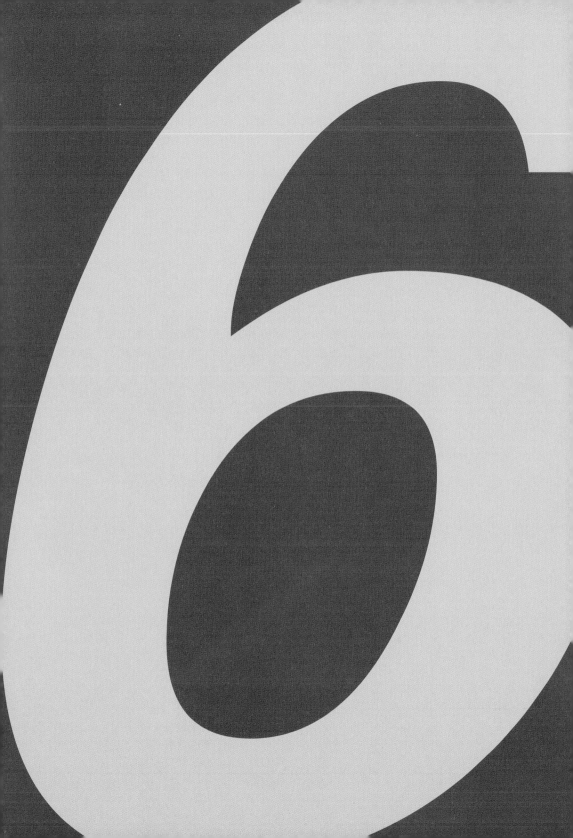

6

Belly Best
Foods List

The following list is for those of you with a strong desire for options outside of the Fast Track Menu in Chapter 4. This list is intended only for substitutions to like items in meals using the Fast Track Menu as your guide. Please refer to the Quick Guidelines on page 85 if you have questions about portion size.

BELLY BEST FOODS

Nuts

Almonds	Hazelnuts	Pistachios
Brazil nuts	Macadamia nuts	Walnuts
	Pecans	

Restorative Proteins

Abalone	Beef shank	Clams
Ahi	Bison	Cod
Anchovies	Bologna	Corned beef
Arctic char	Bratwurst	Cornish game hen
Bacon	Brisket	Crab
Barramundi	Canadian bacon	Deli meat
Bass	Catfish	Duck breast
Beef	Caviar	Duck deli meat
Beef chuck	Chicken breast	Duck thighs
Beef flank	Chicken deli meat	Duck wings
Beef loin	Chicken thighs	Eel
Beef round	Chicken wings	Eggs (any style)

Restorative Proteins (continued)

Escargot	Pepperoni	Spam
Flounder	Pheasant	Squid
Goose	Pollock	Steak
Grouper	Pork	Swordfish
Halibut	Pork loin	Tempeh (only if you're a vegetarian)
Ham	Poultry	
Ham hocks	Primal Fuel meal-replacement shake	Tenderloin
Herring		Tilapia
Hot dog	Quail	Tofu (only if you're a vegetarian)
Jay Robb protein shake	Rabbit	
Jerky	Ribs	Tongue
Lamb	Roast beef	Top sirloin
Liver	Roe	Trout
Lobster	Salami	Tuna
Mackerel	Salmon	Turkey breast
Mahi mahi	Sardines	Turkey deli meat
Mortadella	Sausage	Turkey dogs
Mussels	Scallops	Turkey legs
Mutton	Shark	Turkey wings
Octopus	Shrimp	Veal
Ostrich	Sirloin	Venison
Oysters	Snapper	Wild game
Pastrami	Sole	Yellowtail

Seasonings and Condiments

Alfredo sauce (sugar free)	Cinnamon	Soy sauce (use sparingly)
Allspice	Coriander	Spearmint
Almond extract	Garlic	Tabasco
Almond flour	Ginger	Taco sauce
Anise seed	Horseradish	Tarragon
Basil	Jalapeños	Thyme
Bay leaf	Mayonnaise (sugar free)	Tomatoes (use sparingly)
Black pepper	Mustard	Turmeric
Blackened seasoning	Onions (use sparingly)	Vanilla extract
Capers	Parsley	Vinegar (red wine and apple cider are ideal)
Cayenne powder	Peppermint	
Chives	Pickles (unsweetened)	Wasabi
Cilantro	Shallots	Worcestershire sauce

Good Fats

85% dark chocolate	Brazil nuts	Colby cheese
Almond butter	Brie cheese	Cottage cheese (not fat-free or low-fat)
Almond milk (unsweetened)	Butter	
	Camembert cheese	Cream
Almonds	Cheddar cheese	Cream cheese
American cheese	Coconut milk (unsweetened)	Edam cheese
Avocado		Feta cheese
Blue cheese	Coconut oil	Fish oil

Good Fats (continued)

Flax oil

Fontina cheese

Goat cheese (ideal
for dairy intolerant)

Gouda cheese

Greek yogurt (use
sparingly)

Gruyère cheese

Half-and-half

Heavy cream

Hemp milk

Lard

Limburger cheese

Macadamia nuts

Monterey Jack cheese

Muenster cheese

Neufchâtel cheese

Nuts (also an ideal protein
for vegetarians)

Olive oil

Parmesan cheese

Pecans

Pistachios

Provolone cheese

Sour cream

Walnuts

Whipping cream

Snacks

Black olives

Celery sticks with almond
butter

Cottage cheese topped
with a serving of nuts

Cucumber slices w/
sea salt

Greek yogurt (use
sparingly)

Green olives

Hard-boiled egg

Jay Robb protein shake

Nuts, 1–2 palm-size
servings

Pumpkin seeds

Sandwich meat

String or waxed cheese

Sunflower seeds

Tuna, 1 can

Super Carbs

Alfalfa sprouts

Artichoke hearts (super
high fiber)

Arugula

Asparagus

Bamboo shoots

Bell peppers

Bok choy

Broccoli (super high fiber)

Brussels sprouts (high
fiber)

Super Carbs (continued)

Cabbage	Heart of palm	Sauerkraut (unpasteurized)
Cauliflower	Kale	
Celery	Kimchi (unpasteurized)	Seaweed (high fiber)
Celery root	Leek	Spinach
Chard	Lettuce	Squash, spaghetti
Chicory greens	Mixed greens	Squash, summer
Chicory root	Mushrooms	Squash, winter (high fiber)
Collard greens (high fiber)	Okra (high fiber)	Swiss chard (high fiber)
Cucumber	Onions (use sparingly)	Tomato (use sparingly)
Dill weed	Peppers	Turnip greens
Eggplant	Pickles (unsweetened)	Turnips (high fiber)
Endive	Radicchio	Water chestnuts
Fennel	Radishes	Watercress
		Zucchini

For Vegetarians and Vegans (proteins and fats)

Almond butter	Hazelnuts	Pumpkin seeds
Almonds	Hemp protein shake	Sunflower seeds
Brazil nuts	Macadamia nuts	Tempeh
Chia seeds	Pea protein shake	Tofu
Flax oil	Pecans	Walnuts
	Pistachios	

Nature's Candy		
Apricot (1 medium)	Grapefruit (½ medium)	Pear (½)
Banana (⅓)	Grapes (no raisins, ¼ cup)	Pineapple (¼ cup)
Blackberries (½ cup)		Raspberries (½ cup)
Blueberries (¼ cup)	Mango (¼)	Strawberries (3)
Cantaloupe (⅛)	Nectarine (½ small)	Watermelon (½ cup)
Cherries (not dried, ¼ cup)	Orange (½ small)	

If you are a veteran of the Belly Fat Cure, you probably noticed the reintroduction of fruit. Yes, our good (yet misunderstood) friend fruit is back. Something has changed about him, though. He's not the super-healthy breakfast, snack, juice, or garnish that we always thought he was. In fact, I'm putting our old friend in the candy category.

That's right . . . fruit is candy! Nature's candy, to be exact.

As long as your goal is to lose weight, I recommend eating only very small amounts of fruit. The low-sugar fruits that I recommend as least detrimental to your weight loss are as follows, listed in order of most ideal to least ideal: **raspberries, blackberries, strawberries, blueberries.**

By staying within the list of Belly Best Foods contained in this book, you'll be rewarded with one serving of approved fruit daily as your treat at the end of each day (please refer to Guideline 6 on page 69). And note that I have provided the serving size for each of the fruits in the Belly Best Foods list above.

> *Fruit:*
> *Otherwise known as "nature's candy," it is the most nutritious and natural sweet treat out there. However, large amounts are not ideal for weight loss because of the sugar content.*

7

Conquering an Addiction
to Sugar

"Everything that happens happens as it should, and if you observe carefully, you will find this to be so . . ."

— MARCUS AURELIUS

I've gone to great lengths to expose all the saboteurs you may encounter along your way to a healthy weight and lifestyle. Misinformation and hidden sugar disguised as healthy food can certainly cause you to trip along the way, but what if something more powerful is working against you?

**What if someone in your life wants you
to remain a slave to sugar?**

No, it isn't a family member or a co-worker who wants you to be fat so that he or she has company, although I recommend being prepared for that scenario as well. Rather, your worst enemy may in fact be a part of *yourself.*

Sugar holds great power due to its narcotic nature, and there is the possibility that part of you has become dependent on it over the years . . . the same part of you that surfaces to sabotage your attempts at weight loss. If you have ever felt that *you are your own worst enemy* when it comes to weight loss, then this chapter is for you.

The topic of addiction can be a bit sticky. Some think of it in terms of being a disease, while others shy away from the label because they perceive it to be "an excuse" or an admission of weakness. I don't happen to believe that addiction is any of the above, nor should you be ashamed if you feel powerless at times.

There are many external stimuli people use in order to cope with past pain or current stress, but sugar is by far the most socially acceptable and pervasive. These stimuli—which can include drugs, alcohol, gambling, shopping, work, or even sex—all distract you from a feeling you don't want to feel. Taboo and undesirable as the topic of emotional pain may be, I would be cheating you if I did not include it in this book for one crucial reason:

No matter what you eat or how much you exercise,
you will remain sick and overweight if you
use food to numb emotional pain.

I certainly don't assume that you are an emotional eater; that is for you to decide. But how can you tell? Ask yourself these questions:

- Do you seek comfort in food when you're sad?

- Do you often continue to eat, even after feeling "stuffed"?

- Do you often eat out of boredom?

- Do you feel compelled to eat the most food at night, before bed?

- Have you ever felt as if you have no control over your choices?

If you answered "Yes" to two or more of these questions, then you may sometimes use food to cope. The first step is just to recognize that fact. If you did answer "Yes" to two or more questions, I'd like you to say the following, either aloud or just to yourself: "Sometimes I eat to escape my feelings." Admit it, own it, and don't be ashamed of it. "Sometimes I eat to escape my feelings."

Guess what? I still love you! Your friends and family still love you! And if you can just accept love from *yourself,* the pain of emotional eating will begin to heal. Much like a probiotic treats not just the symptoms but also the cause of digestive problems, you must reach deep inside to replace the fear and pain with a sense of self-worth and nurturing practices that will remove your dependence on harmful external stimuli to cope.

I want to share all this with you because I myself was an emotional eater, and this is really a journey you and I are on together. At the end of our road is not only better health and a smaller size, but also our greatest potential.

The Path to Addiction

If we were all born with the genetic potential to be healthy and happy, how did we end up *here?* The answer, I believe, is that here is exactly where we need to be. No matter your weight, health, financial situation, or relationship status, *here* is the only place you can *learn* the lessons and *meet* the people and *change* the lives you must. Whether you view that through religion, logic, or spirituality, the following remains true:

**You can only succeed at shaping your future
if you accept your past and present.**

Once you have forgiven yourself for whatever blame you may be carrying, it's time to discover the source of your fear. Whether you care to admit it or not, you have fear. We all do. But each and every one of us also has love. Despite the wide range of emotions we experience, they are all merely varying degrees of two primal emotions: fear and love. This has hardly changed over the course of history, but what has changed is how we deal with the fear-based emotions we feel: we either numb them or try to escape them rather than acknowledge and work through them.

Thanks to the proliferation and social acceptance of processed sugar and starchy comfort foods, we have access to a completely legal and stigma-free sedative at all times. The reliance may begin as a means to escape from childhood experiences such as tragedy, abuse, trauma, neglect, teasing, or rejection. Most of us have been subjected to several of these experiences before even reaching those turbulent middle- and high-school years. Our coping mechanism soothes the pain we feel, and before long we're reaching for it to help us endure smaller and smaller problems.

Fast-forward 10 or 20 years, and the emotional "muscle" needed to survive even the most tranquil life has completely atrophied. Anything and everything unpleasant sparks an intense desire to escape, including the very consequences of using the coping mechanism. The shame of being overweight as a result of using sugar to cope makes one want to, you guessed it, eat more sugar.

This is why addiction is never in neutral.
It is a fire that creates its own fuel.

But what provided the first spark? For most people, feelings of inadequacy originate from the way they were treated by their primary caregivers. There are two ways in which most self-worth issues arise: overdependence and over*in*dependence.

Our primary caregivers may have treated us in a way that made us feel overly dependent on them and unsure of our own abilities. Consequently, we were left feeling helpless, overprotected, smothered, and incapable. For instance, my grandmother,

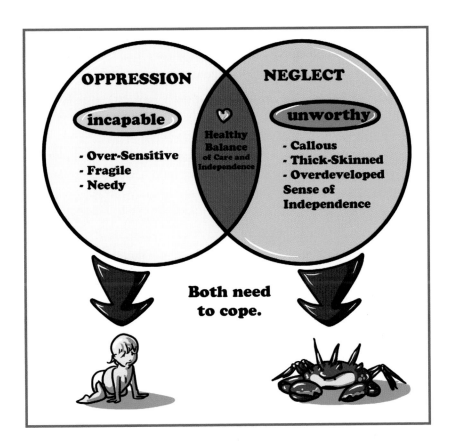

bless her heart, did the very best she knew how to when raising me. The moment I cried, there was a bottle in my mouth. But she also told me that I was too *"delicado"* and the world was too dangerous for me. I was conditioned to believe that I was completely dependent on others.

To this day I dearly love my *abuelita,* and I feel blessed that she was my primary caregiver. I realize that she didn't deliberately intend to cause harm to me, and that she was acting in a way that she considered to be protective and loving. But in response to her overly protective nature, I developed dependent behavior patterns that are not effective as an adult. I chose to acknowledge my ineffective behavior patterns and to work at replacing that dependency with the strength and confidence that is essential for maintaining healthy relationships as an adult.

When you're as closely guarded as I was, you end up with an overly developed sense of **dependence on others.** You become hypersensitive, like someone without skin; even the slightest touch is extremely painful. On top of lacking any kind of emotional defense, the original feelings of inadequacy are hard to shake. I was fat, sick, and addicted to sugar as a child because it numbed me, making me feel less weak and pathetic. It numbed me until it almost killed me when my appendix unexpectedly burst at the age of 14.

On the flip side, our primary caregivers may have treated us in a way that made us feel neglected. We feel as though we have no one to rely on other than ourselves, and seek to live in a world in which all of our needs are met strictly through our own actions. Then, as young people, we have an overly developed sense of **independence from others.** In such an individualistic society, we tend to highly value qualities like independence. No doubt, many incredibly successful and driven people arose from situations of neglect or even abuse.

However, life is not an individual sport. Relying on others is an inherent part of our human nature, but it is suppressed in people who had to grow up very quickly and become completely independent in order to survive. These individuals *fear* relying on others, and have an emotional skin that is completely calloused over because they're too afraid to feel. They appear tough and in control, but the neglect of their childhood and resulting aversion to getting close to anyone makes them feel unworthy of love and unable to feel truly connected to others. Desperate to escape deep feelings, they are often very lonely.

The result is that two different people from two completely opposite circumstances arrive at the same destination: both with no sense of self-worth and with coping skills that now hinder their potential as adults. Their coping mechanisms from their difficult childhoods are still their default solutions to fear, even if and when they leave the unhealthy situation behind (by going to college, for instance). New stress enters their lives in the form of exams, finances, relationships, career choices, and breakups; and the dependency on external stimuli to escape grows.

Protect and Nurture to Heal Your Life

I wish I could say the strategy that replaced my own coping mechanisms with the nurturing that helped me heal is "just three simple steps"! But that would fail to do justice to what can be a very long and painful process. I won't try to downplay the journey toward emotional healing, but I will tell you that it's definitely a road worth traveling.

Know that if you follow these steps, you absolutely can heal your life:

- **Protect** yourself from triggers, compulsions, and escapes

- **Nurture** the growth of your emotional strength

- **Heal** your life by creating a compelling future

The first step is to simply protect yourself from immediate danger, which means knowing exactly what to do when your compulsion is trying to drag you to the pantry around midnight. When the urge to escape from sadness or stress using food (or alcohol or shopping or what have you) first appears, I want you to use any or all of the following four strategies:

1. Breathing. The easiest entry-level practice to protect your body from a compulsion is as simple as breathing deeply. Eastern medicine has viewed breathing as "the emotional digestive system" for thousands of years, and you'll understand why after just a few short minutes of practice.

The trick is to perform what is known in yoga as **Ujjayi** breathing, also known as "ocean breath." You breathe deeply and slowly, in and out through the nose, with a

Ujjayi:
An ancient breathing technique that helps quiet the mind and bring one's focus to the breath. Deep breathing such as Ujjayi is the body's "emotional digestive system."

slight contraction in the back of the throat. As your breath rises and falls, it will sound somewhat like the waves of a relatively calm ocean washing ashore. Adding this audible sound to your breath gives you a point of focus as you practice breathing deeply and slowly, returning your body to a calmer, more collected baseline. I recommend anywhere from five minutes to an hour of this practice, always trying to keep your mind from wandering by returning your thoughts to the rise and fall of your breath.

2. Words of empowerment. If you say something enough, you believe it. If you believe something enough, it often comes true. No, I'm not talking about lottery jackpots here, but rather about how your beliefs have a huge impact on your destiny. If you believe you can't do it, then you're right, you can't. It doesn't matter what you eat or how much you exercise because **"I can't do it" is the most consistent self-fulfilling prophecy in the world.**

I talk to people all the time who tell me, "I just can't do it. If I could lose ten pounds, then maybe I'd believe that I could do it. Please tell me what to do to lose those ten pounds!" This really puts the cart before the horse; with such an attitude, I guarantee that those individuals won't lose the ten pounds they've come to believe are the key to their future happiness and health. I won't make even one food recommendation to a client until I can get him or her to say "I *can* do it." Surprisingly, just getting someone to say those words (even without believing them) can be like pulling teeth!

I want you to use words of empowerment to begin shaping your belief system to be more nurturing of your goals. You can do so by simply being your own "cheerleader," even if a lot of what you say feels like you're just pretending at first. Your power words and phrases can be anything you like, spoken in front of a mirror or not, but always said out loud.

Here are some suggestions of wonderful affirmations, or words of empowerment:

I love you.

I can do this.

Wow, you look great!

This is the time I win.

I am beautiful.

I am loved.

Louise Hay, author of the landmark self-help book *You Can Heal Your Life,* developed a great forgiveness exercise that I often share with my clients: every morning when you wake up, look in the mirror, and forgive aloud parts of your body that give you anxiety.

Here is an example that came from one of my own clients:

"Good morning, hips. I love you. I forgive you for not looking like the hips I see on magazine covers. You probably wouldn't be very happy if you looked like that anyway. I still love you, hips. You are beautiful, hips. I'll always forgive you."

It took at least 30 minutes—and a lot of pleading, tough love, and crying—to get this particular woman to face her hips and forgive something she thought had tortured her for decades. The release of that forgiveness was phenomenal.

The bottom line when it comes to power words is this: even if you don't start out believing the things you say, you *will.* Keep saying that you can do it, and you can. Say that you are beautiful, and you will be. The same is true of negative words and phrases. It can be hard to stop beating yourself up after so long, but believing in yourself and using positive words and phrases to rewrite the story of your life is absolutely more important than knowing what to eat.

3. Muscle intensification. This is a great protective measure for whenever cravings, or the underlying feelings that trigger them, pop up. All you have to do is tighten up every muscle in your body for about two seconds and release, and then repeat.

I recommend assuming the fetal position as you squeeze every muscle in your body as tightly as you can. Squeeze, relax, repeat. Squeeze, relax, repeat. Like many things in this book, it can sound a little goofy at first, but it really works. Try just 20 repetitions the next time you sense anxiety stirring, preferably before it turns into a full-blown craving or a compulsion to escape from that anxiety.

4. Eye-movement therapy. If you thought my last recommendation sounded bizarre, then you'll really love this one! Eye Movement Desensitization and Reprocessing (EMDR) is a form of psychotherapy originally developed in the late '80s by Francine Shapiro to help people cope with traumatic memories, including those suffering from post-traumatic stress disorder (PTSD).

My version of eye-movement therapy is based on similar concepts as EMDR and may alleviate just about any painful memory from which you seek relief. In my opinion, this technique is best when performed with the help of someone you love and trust, but it can be done alone. (*Please note:* while I feel that self-help is a great alternative for many people, I do urge you to seek treatment with a medical or mental-health provider if indicated for any specific condition.)

Here is how to perform the eye-movement-therapy exercise, step-by-step:

— Focus on the memory from which you seek relief, and boil down the experience to one image. It is preferable to focus on an image that you believe encapsulates the most traumatic point of your experience.

— Create a belief statement by asking yourself, *What words about myself or the incident best go with the picture?* The statement should really reflect how the incident made you feel, perhaps something like *I am helpless, I should have done something,* or *I have no control.* These are just examples, and the statement must accurately reflect your own feelings of the traumatic experience.

— While both visualizing the traumatic image from the first step and rehearsing the statement or feeling associated with the trauma from the second step, hold your finger (or have a partner hold his or her finger) about 12 to 14 inches from your eyes. Focus on the finger and move it rhythmically back and forth across the line of vision from the far right to the far left, with about two back-and-forth movements per second. Move the eyes to track the finger, but keep the head completely still. One set is about 12 seconds long.

— At the end of the set, erase the image from your mind and take a deep breath. At the end of the breath, pull up the same image and the associated belief and begin the exercise again.

You may think this all sounds too easy, but according to one study, traumatized subjects found that with each new round, it became more and more difficult to pull up the traumatic image. They also found it harder to believe or accept completely the statement they had associated with the image. Many were led to other traumas they had somehow been unaware of, or other beliefs they needed to overcome but had been unable to admit. Categorically, the subjects managed to desensitize themselves to the traumatic experience and the associated belief, which is another way of saying they released the power the trauma had over them.

I recommend doing ten sets of my eye-movement exercise whenever anxiety, doubt, or feelings of self-loathing creep in. And if you're carrying the effects of trauma (yes, teasing counts!), which must be healed in order for you to move on, I strongly recommend that you perform ten sets of this exercise every night.

Keep in mind that it is important to always reassess the first two steps of the process, so your image and belief statement can change as you make progress through the healing. For example, your statement may begin as *I have no control,* but then progress to *I'm not worthy of love* as the process opens your heart and mind to self-discovery.

Nurture the Growth of Your Emotional Strength

The preceding exercises are great, but there is almost always a deeper healing that is required. The goal of such a healing is to realize that you possess all the love and strength you will ever need inside yourself already. When you call upon your belief that you are worthy of self-love and the love of others, you become free of a dependence on external coping mechanisms and no longer require validation from others. Your ultimate goal is to be able to validate yourself.

There are several practices that can aid in this process, and each is considerably less expensive than seeing a therapist. Dr. Christiane Northrup once gave me the profound advice that we all must "feel it to heal it." It may sound like a great sound bite, but it is truly so much more than that.

When you think about the cause and effect of the emotional side of overeating (or any compulsion), is it the pain that caused the weight gain? At the root, yes, but the more direct cause of overeating is the desire to *escape* from pain. If you commit to feeling the pain instead of trying to escape it, you throw a wrench into the cycle that nourishes your compulsive eating. "Feel it" can mean grieving for something that feels lost or forgiving someone or something you think wronged you, or it can be anything that upsets you. It depends completely on your individual experience.

The bottom line here is to stop being such a trouper, and cry it out! You get no bonus points for the tears you manage to hold back; I'd even argue that those unrealized tears poison you. The same is true of old grudges and hurt feelings that you hold on to. Whoever it was that called you names in the third grade doesn't deserve any of the power you continue to give him or her by allowing those words to affect your sense of self-worth *now.* It sounds simple, but I know all too well just how difficult that first act of forgiveness and release can be. Trust me . . . the payoff is so much more rewarding than that first step is scary.

Heal Your Life by Creating a Compelling Future

Another exercise I love and practice myself is a future diary, because nothing is a more powerful motivator than a **compelling future.** This can even be a really fun activity that you can do with your kids, and they'll never know that "playtime" is actually therapeutic.

All you have to do is get a journal or notebook and create your ideal future. This future can be six months, a year, or five years from now—or however far into the future you want to go—but you must make it as compelling as possible. Don't spare any details. I also strongly recommend using images in your future diary because pictures and symbols tend to have more power than words. You can go through old magazines and cut out images, search online, or draw your own.

> **Compelling future:**
> A positive event that could occur in the future if you make the right choices. This event or outcome should be so attractive that it is a powerful motivator to make the right choices as often as you can.

When I meet people who "can't do it," the one thing they all have in common is that they lack a compelling future. The only future they've created for themselves (in their mind) is one where they end up "fat and alone," and that isn't much to look forward to. It's also another example of a self-fulfilling prophecy.

Imagine yourself dancing at your daughter's wedding and being the life of the party at the reception. By creating that future on paper, you get a taste of how you would feel in that moment . . . and it's so sweet! These feelings and images motivate you to do positive things like walk in the morning and swap that sugary "blueberry" muffin for eggs instead. If you picture a future in which you're unloved, you won't be able to make the right choices when it counts.

Finally, just as you created a future diary, I recommend creating a **Dickens diary.** Remember the Charles Dickens classic *A Christmas Carol,* where the ghosts of Christmases past, present, and future visit Ebenezer Scrooge? This diary is like that, only with fewer ghosts. Using words and images, create a story about how using your particular crutch (food, shopping, or the like) has affected your life. What consequences has it had in the past, what consequences does it have now, and what consequences could it have in the future if you don't stop using it?

Maybe you don't make it to your daughter's wedding, and instead she gives a tearful toast wishing you were there to see her in her beautiful dress. Spend just ten minutes depicting in as much detail as possible that exact moment in your daughter's future and you may never look at sugary coping foods in the same way again.

When you put your compelling future next to your Dickens diary, the price of relying on external sources to numb pain becomes painfully crystal clear. Take your new art projects and put them on the wall or fridge in your home as a reminder of why the foods you put in your mouth are so important.

You Are Already Loved

I have done a lot of research into what my clients want. Not just what they *say* they want (health) but what they *really* want (love). As a society, we've all been conditioned by advertising to believe that once we look a certain way, we will be loved. Considering the fact that being loved is just as important as food and shelter, this method of advertising motivates us remarkably well. However, it is another example of the cart before the horse.

You won't receive love once you lose weight,
**YOU WILL LOSE WEIGHT
ONCE YOU RECEIVE LOVE!**

I wish I could follow that completely true statement with the world's biggest smiley face. You must believe you are loved, and accept that love, especially from yourself. Release the blame, because it isn't your fault. Forgive your parents and your exes. Look yourself in the eye and tell yourself that you *can* do it. Whether you follow my food plan or not, please take this advice. I lived so much of my life feeling unworthy of everything good I had—because even good things feel meaningless when you don't love yourself. If anything in your past or present makes you feel as though you can relate, and you would like to join me on the other side, the exercises in this chapter will get you there.

How do I know that you are already loved? Because here you are, participating in what is truly my life's work. For that fact, *I* love you. You have the ability to take my dream and make it real. You have the ability to change the world you live in, all by simply living your best life and setting an example for the people around you. I sincerely hope that every single one of you who reads this book and experiences its life-changing effects will reach out and share this knowledge with your mother, father, sons, daughters, aunts, uncles, and everyone else around you. It is my dream that you will take an active part in the revolution that must occur to stop the tide of obesity and disease that threatens us all.

Please visit and join me in my dream of seeing 30 million people awaken from the myths that hold us all back. Whether you share something you found helpful with three friends, or simply cook a delicious low-sugar meal that your family can't believe is healthy, you will have done something so powerful and so important. Inspiring you to make and share this change is what I believe to be my purpose on this earth.

For your help, I love you more than you will ever know.

FAST TRACK
SUCCESS STORY

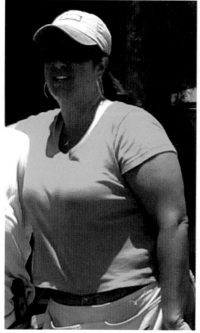

Before

Age: 43
Height: 5'7"
Pounds Lost: 28

I've always been grateful for the amazing things I have in life, as well as being very vocal about "seizing the day" to my close circle of friends. Deep down, though, I also wondered if people could take me seriously . . . if I had control of my life and was truly happy, then why was I overweight?

Jorge revealed to me the part deep inside that I've been hiding from the rest of the world. Thanks to the tools and motivation he's given me, I've taken charge over that final part of my life in need of a little TLC. For the first time ever, I feel like my outside is reflecting how I feel on the inside, and I want to share my joy with the people I love now more than ever. Look out, world, no more excuses! It's time for me to stop hiding and start living!

My new attitude is also helped by probably the most important benefit I've personally experienced on this program: I can sleep through the night! Troubled sleep has been a drag on my life for as long as I can remember, and the first thing I noticed within a few days of the Fast Track program was the most restful sleep I'd ever known. So for anyone out there who feels like they're never able to reach their full potential because they're never able to feel rested, you must try this program. It changed my life, and I know it will change yours, too!

Andrea
Lost 28 pounds!

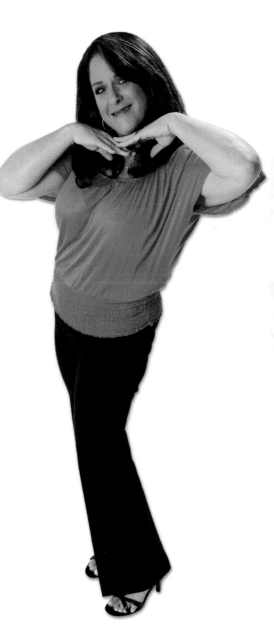

What's Next?

People tend to work on their outsides and neglect what is on the inside. Now that I know how to eat to continue to look and feel great, I've turned my attention to the things that really matter. I'm crossing "weight loss" off my list for good, and making a new list of more important things I want to accomplish in life!

My Best Tip

Don't think about losing weight as strictly an issue of looking better. Following through with this program means that you'll have so much more love to share with the people you care about! And believe me, that love makes its way back to you.

FAST TRACK SUCCESS STORY

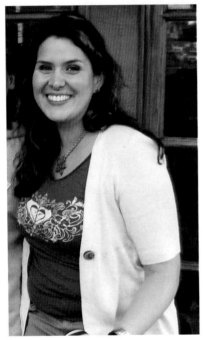

Before

Age: 35
Height: 5'8"
Pounds Lost: 15

Before starting the Fast Track program, I suffered from debilitating migraines and had been on pain medications and steroids to manage them. I also had continuous back and neck pain as the result of a car accident seven years ago. Now I am much more active and feel great! I've only had one migraine, and it came on immediately after eating a processed hot dog and washing it down with a diet cola. My neurologist has been working with me and tracking my progress and has been very supportive of my new eating habits.

On top of those wonderful health benefits, I feel like I look great everywhere I go now! When I was younger I competed in beauty pageants, and I remember walking on the stage with confidence and presence. I had almost completely forgotten what that felt like over the years as I slowly put on weight and felt sluggish from the chronic pain I experienced as a result of my accident. Whenever I walk into a room now, I feel like Miss Chula Vista all over again. My self-confidence is back, baby!

Ali
Lost 15 pounds!

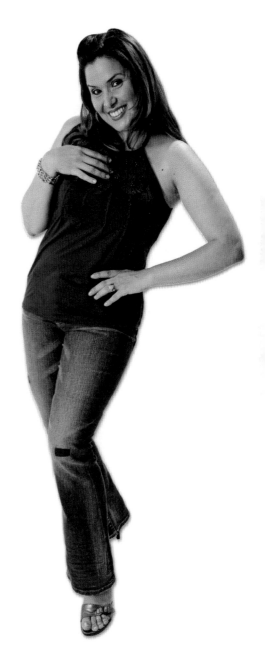

What's Next?

Now that my health is back on track, it has freed up my time and energy to live my life and focus my attention on joyful things like my family and my art. For the first time I also feel like I have the health and energy to start a family of my own, something I just never had the confidence to do before the Fast Track.

My Best Tip

Having my husband, Karl (page 198), live the Fast Track lifestyle with me has been invaluable. We have truly enjoyed learning about how these foods affect our health, and we love cooking and shopping at Costco together. We love to encourage each other and spend so much more quality time doing activities like hiking and biking. Succeeding on this program has completely transformed our marriage and helped us build even more trust and intimacy that has brought joy back into our lives!

FAST TRACK
SUCCESS
STORY

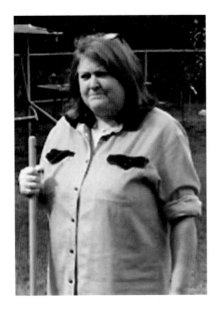

Before

Age: 55
Height: 5'0"
Pounds Lost: 28

Now that I've been following the Fast Track program, my energy level has increased 100 percent. I feel better and am able to exercise again without the pain and shortness of breath I used to experience. I enjoy cooking every night now and eating lots of healthy food, as opposed to wasting money on all that tasteless junk I used to rely on.

My whole family has changed dramatically in the way that we interact with each other because of our new commitment to health. We enjoy the process of preparing food together and actually sitting down and deliberately sharing a meal together, getting healthier with each bite. I even went and got my blood work done, and my triglycerides have dropped from 232 to 177 during the weeks since I adopted this lifestyle.

It wasn't long ago that my husband, Chris (page 42), and I wondered if we were going to be around to enjoy our girls as they grew up. Now we're looking forward to the future with an enthusiasm and excitement we haven't felt in years. Jorge and his team helped us redefine our future, and it has changed our family tree for generations to come. We are truly blessed to have been on the Fast Track program together.

Sue
Lowered triglycerides by 55!

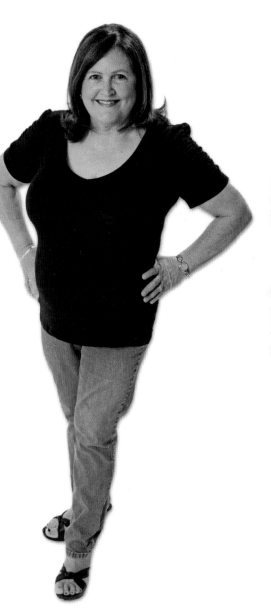

What's Next?

One of the side benefits our family discovered while on the Fast Track was a love for cooking. It has been an amazing bonding experience, and I've uncovered a true passion for making family-pleasing meals that I never thought I could before. I plan on continuing to use my skills and creativity with all the Belly Best Foods to continue to grow my new talent!

My Best Tip

There is strength in two or more people working together to achieve a goal. Everyone needs support. Whether it's made up of friends, family, co-workers, or other followers of the Belly Fat Cure, build yourself a team if you want to guarantee success!

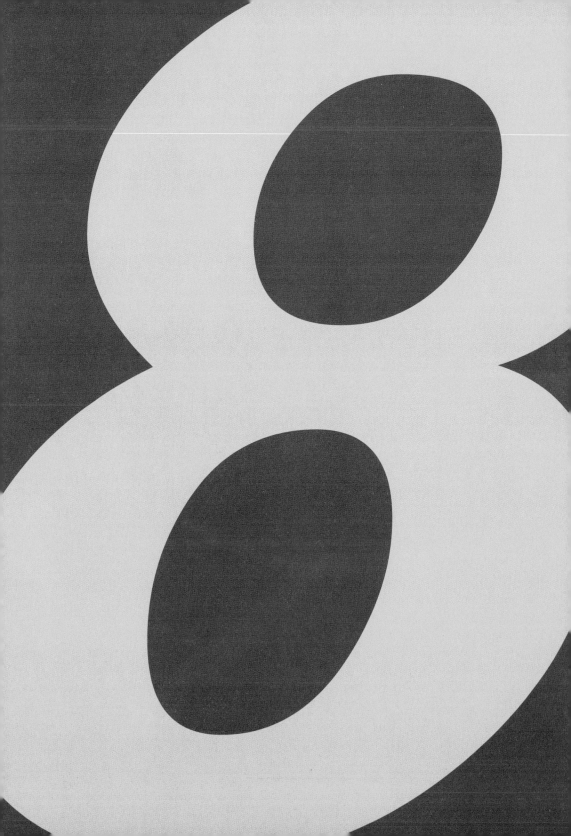

Simply Fit™:
Burn Belly Fat

"High-intensity intermittent exercise results in greater fat loss directly in the abdomen."

— DR. STEPHEN BOUTCHER

When it comes to exercise, quality is more important than quantity. Exercising in short bursts of activity—known as high-intensity interval training (HIIT), or high-intensity intermittent exercise—actually allows you to exercise less while burning more fat than regular workouts! In a groundbreaking study published in the *International Journal of Obesity,* researchers found that women who did 20-minute sessions of HIIT 3 times a week lost more subcutaneous fat and improved their insulin resistance more than the group who exercised at a continuous, moderate pace for twice as long.

Dr. Stephen Boutcher, an esteemed expert on obesity and one of the researchers in the study, says that "numerous scientific studies do not support spot fat reduction." In other words, exercise causes fat from all over the body to be reduced, not just the areas you want to target. He points to elite tennis players to demonstrate this concept. If spot-reduction exercise were effective, he says, a player's racket arm should contain much less fat. However, researchers have shown that the while the racket arms of tennis players usually possess greater muscle and bone mass, both arms have similar levels of fat.

Numerous studies by Dr. Boutcher prove that HIIT is "more effective at reducing subcutaneous and abdominal body fat than other types of exercise." The visceral fat that surrounds your organs is also known as "killer fat" because it is directly linked to poor health outcomes. Visceral fat has greater blood flow, so it is even more responsive to belly-fat loss than subcutaneous fat, which is located just under the skin.

HOW TO BE SIMPLY FIT™

So here's what your HIIT routine will look like: you'll be alternating between 2 moves for 20 minutes, 3 days a week. After a 3-minute warm-up of your choice, you'll do a high-intensity move for 8 seconds, then an active-recovery move for 12 seconds, repeating for a full 20 minutes with no break. Follow this with a 3-minute cool down, and that's it—you're done! Your body will be burning fat for hours and hours to come.

Your 8-second intervals are high-intensity, full-body moves designed to get your heart pumping. These are explosive movements that you'll be able to sustain for only a short time before moving on to the 12-second active-recovery exercise. In active recovery, you'll be focusing on strength and endurance as opposed to cardio. Your heart rate should drop a bit so you can catch your breath, but you should still be working hard rather than resting. It will be tough, but this is your chance to spur your body to open up the fat-burning floodgates!

Over the next few pages, you'll find 6 options for your 8- and 12-second intervals that you can combine to create a simple, at-home routine. For even more variety in a fun, engaging, high-energy environment, please visit JorgeCruise.com.

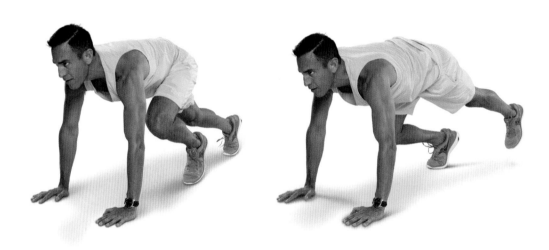

8-Second Interval: Mountain Climber

Start in push-up position on hands and toes. Keeping your hips low and your head in line with your spine, bring one knee toward your chest in a fluid motion. Return foot to starting position, then bring in other knee. Alternate sides as quickly as possible.

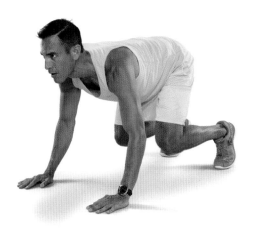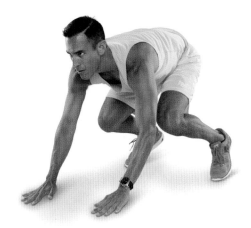

12-Second Interval: Frog Push-up

Start on the floor in push-up position, hands hip-distance apart with your fingers pointing forward. Bend your elbows slightly, and move your feet closer to your hands so your legs are bent at a 90-degree angle, keeping your knees and heels off the floor. With your weight on your toes and palms, shift your weight forward and lower only your upper body until your nose is close to the ground, then push back up.

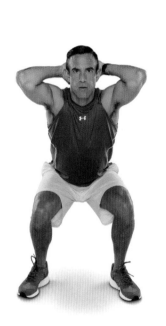
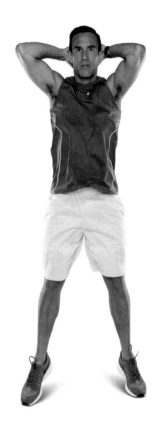

8-Second Interval: Squat Jumps

Place feet shoulder-width apart, hands behind your head with your elbows forward. Lower yourself until your hips are at or below your knees, and hold this position for a second. Then jump up as high as you can. Repeat.

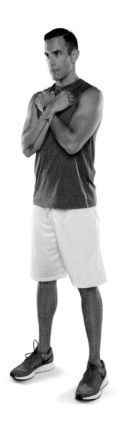
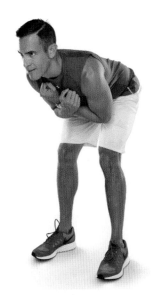

12-Second Interval: Hip Hinges

Stand with feet shoulder-width apart and arms across your chest. Shift your weight to your heels and push your hips back, bending your knees slightly, as you bend your torso forward to about a 45-degree angle. Contract your glutes as you stand up. Repeat.

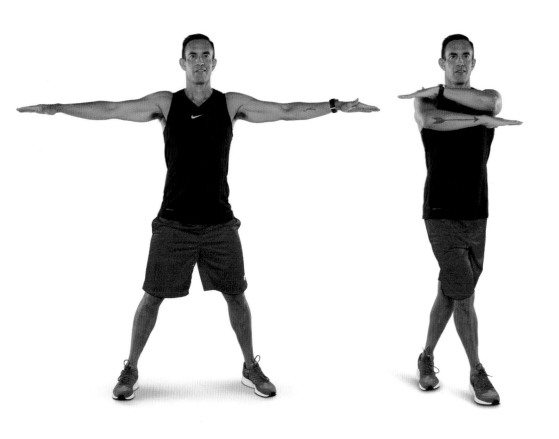

8-Second Interval: Cross Jacks

Stand with your feet shoulder-width apart and extend your arms straight out to either side with palms facing down. Jump and place your right foot over your left while swinging both arms in to cross your right arm over your left. Jump back to the starting position, then jump again to cross with the opposite arm and foot. Quickly continue alternating sides.

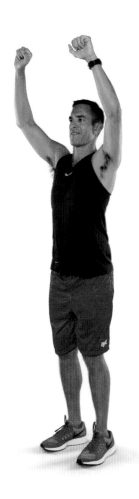
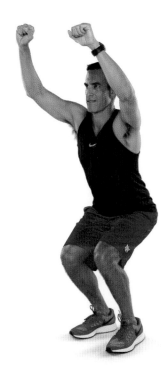

12-Second Interval: Deep Overhead Squat

Stand with your feet hip-width apart, toes pointing outward slightly, and arms raised above your head. Keep your back straight and head up as you lower yourself down, pushing your hips back and bending your knees, until your thighs are parallel with the ground. (Be sure to initiate the movement with your hips, and don't let your knees move forward beyond your toes.) Return to standing position by extending your knees, hips, and ankles. Come to a fully erect position before lowering into the next repetition.

FAST TRACK
SUCCESS
STORY

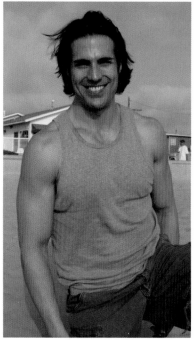

Before

Age: 40
Height: 5'11"
Pounds Lost: 10

As a former fashion and fitness model, I've always had to put a lot of time, effort, and pain into staying in top shape. Then about a year ago, I decided that I wanted to get bigger and more muscular. For anyone out there who has tried to put on a lot of muscle, you know that bodybuilders will always tell you one thing: you have to eat lots of carbs! Since pretty much everyone in the industry was telling me this, I didn't question it. I worked out hard and ate lots of carbs I thought were healthy, like brown rice, just like I'd been told.

All my weight lifting paid off and I did put on a good amount of muscle, but at a price. Slowly but surely, my six-pack turned into a two-pack. It seemed like every time I looked in the mirror, I was more and more puffy. Again, all my body-building friends told me, "That's just the way it is," and I believed there just wasn't any other way to build muscle without also gaining fat.

Then I met Jorge here in San Diego, and he changed my perspective entirely. I learned that fat is the ideal source of energy, and that avoiding saturated fat wasn't a strategy for getting ripped like I'd been told. He also clued me in to the ideal source of carbohydrates: nutrient-packed green vegetables he liked to call Super

Julian
Lost 10 pounds!

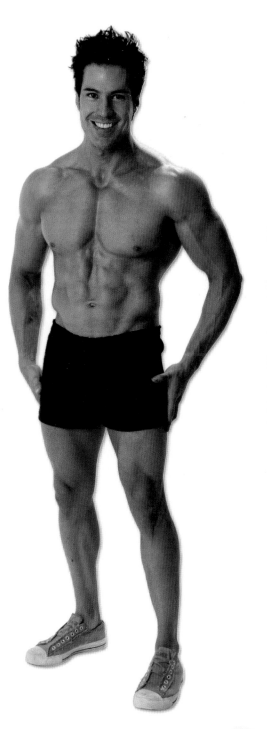

Carbs. Luckily for me, I'd been avoiding simple sugars all my life because I knew that they'd affect my physique. Now that Jorge has shared with me how sugar causes aging, I avoid the stuff like the plague!

What's Next?

I'm always looking to improve my physique in order to land new jobs, and Jorge's recommendations have helped me do just that. I feel better than ever, and have way more energy to hit the gym . . . which is basically my place of business. I've never been this big and this cut in my life before, and it rocks!

My Best Tip

This is a tip for all the guys out there trying to pack on some hard muscle: fat will help your muscles grow just as well as carbs, without getting that carby, bloated look. So put down the brown rice and leave those yolks in your omelette!

FAST TRACK
SUCCESS STORY

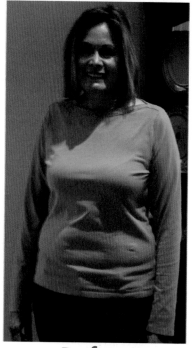

Before

Age: 57
Height: 5'8"
Pounds Lost: 20

After retiring, I put on about 20 pounds. More bothersome than the weight was the fact that I was always tired! Here I was, free to do whatever I wanted and enjoy the rewards of a life of hard work, and I was just too tired to take advantage of it. My clothes didn't fit, I was getting crankier with each passing day, and my hubby wasn't afraid to let me know that he'd noticed a difference. Well, thank goodness for that!

Now that I've done the Fast Track program, I hardly ever have cravings or feel hungry—all while eating healthier, more enjoyable meals. Not only do my clothes fit better, but my mind is sharper and my energy is through the roof! And as for my hubby, he still can't decide which he likes more: the fact that I'm not cranky anymore or that he has 20 fewer pounds to carry on the back of his Harley!

This new way of eating is so easy that anyone can do it. There are so many good foods to choose from, and I especially enjoy eating at restaurants guilt free. The fact that hidden sugar is truly poison is something I believe everyone should know about. I can honestly walk around the grocery store and my craving for sweets is gone, which is a miracle. Thanks, Jorge!

Gloria
Lost 20 pounds!

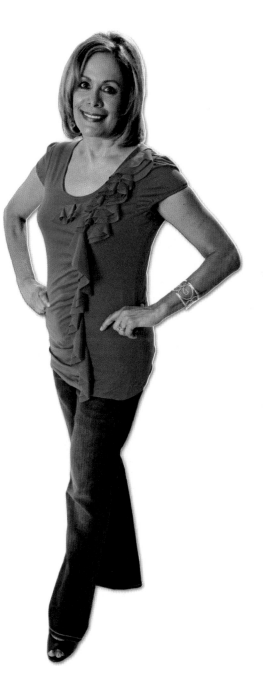

What's Next?

With better health and the more positive outlook that has come with it, I can really focus on squeezing as much joy from each day of these golden years as possible. I look forward to cruising the open road on the back of my hubby's Harley with more confidence and love of life. Now that I know I don't have to stop eating healthy food every time I want to go on a trip, I'm ready to ride on a moment's notice!

My Best Tip

Be prepared to pick yourself up if and when you slip on the program. I "cheated" one night, but I didn't beat myself up about it—I picked up right where I left off the next morning at breakfast. If you can ditch the all-or-nothing approach to weight loss, it becomes much more difficult to create a reason to give up!

FAST TRACK
SUCCESS
STORY

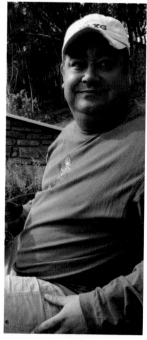

Before

Age: 43
Height: 6'0"
Pounds Lost: 35

Like a lot of the amazing people who started on the Fast Track program with me, I had struggled with weight management for years. I had a condition known as Graves' disease, which caused my thyroid gland to swell up to the size of a ten-ounce steak wrapped around my neck . . . the surgery to remove it nearly ended my life. Without my thyroid, and with my metabolism "out of whack," I thought I had no choice but to be overweight for the rest of my life.

However, after only three weeks of simply eating different food, I felt better than at any point in the last ten years. Also, let me clarify that when I say "different" food, what I mean is *better* food! Not only have I lost weight, but I have higher levels of consistent energy throughout the day, I feel crisp and alert, and I wake up feeling rested without all the aches and pains that I thought were just an inescapable part of being over 40.

Even at 255 pounds, I managed to climb Mt. Whitney, hiked the High Sierra Trail, and planted over 15,000 tree seedlings and counting . . . all things made possible through the support of my amazing family and friends. Now that I'm on the Belly Fat Cure, I look forward to even tougher climbs and to returning all the

Karl
Lost 35 pounds!

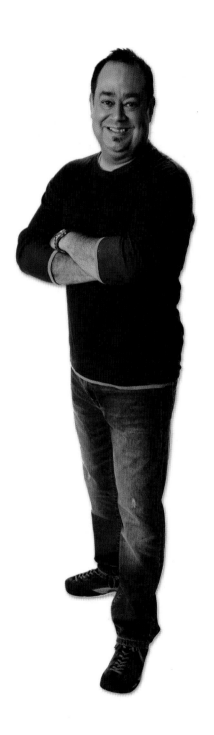

love and support I've been blessed with. Thank you, Jorge and team, for opening my eyes to the life I was meant to live!

What's Next?

My wife, Ali (page 180), and I are planning a Yosemite backpacking trip later this year, which is something we never would have been able to do together without us both overcoming the chronic pains and stiffness that slowed us down. With more energy, I've also devoted even more time to planting seedlings in areas affected by wildfire, a cause that I couldn't be more passionate about.

My Best Tip

Prep your meals and snacks ahead of time, and find a loved one to do the program with. Having my beautiful wife as my partner on the program has kept us both accountable and motivated. We have grown so much closer thanks to this opportunity!

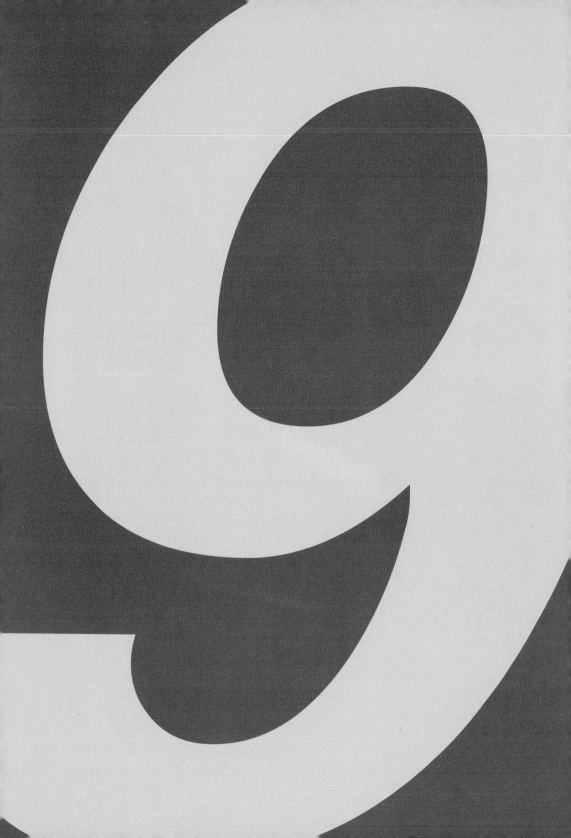

Frequently Asked Questions
FAQs

1. What is the difference between the Belly Fat Cure Fast Track program and Atkins?

Both the Belly Fat Cure Fast Track program and the Atkins Diet focus on carbohydrates to limit insulin production, but the similarities stop there. There are six major distinctions that make the Fast Track program a more healthful, more effective weight-loss accelerator:

— **No ketosis.** The main goal of Atkins is to induce ketosis, which is a state the body enters when it is severely restricted of carbohydrates from all sources. Dieters following Atkins often buy strips that they urinate on to test for ketosis, but you won't ever be doing that on the Belly Fat Cure. Rather than attempting to induce ketosis, we focus on obtaining carbs from the most healthful and easily absorbable sources.

— **No dangerous artificial sweeteners.** Atkins relies heavily on the use of artificial sweeteners like sucralose, while the Belly Fat Cure eliminates this and all other unnatural and potentially harmful chemicals from your diet. Without weaning yourself from the constant stimulation of your sweet tooth, you'll continue to experience cravings that almost always pull you off course. This may be the reason why researchers at the University of Texas Health Science Center at San Antonio found that for every can of diet soda someone had each day, his or her risk of obesity increased by 41 percent!

— **"No carbs" vs. "Super Carbs."** It is important to understand the distinction between "carbs" and the foods that contain them. Atkins makes no distinction between foods rich in carbohydrates and restricts them all. The Fast Track program, however, only restricts those sources (sugar, grains, starches, legumes) that our bodies are poorly adapted to and that have lower nutrient density. You are afforded, even encouraged, to eat carbs on the Fast Track so long as they come from the most ideal and nutrient-rich sources: green vegetables, aka Super Carbs.

— **Alkalinity.** The foods recommended on Atkins fail to factor in one huge health issue: alkalinity. The human body desires an internal environment that is slightly alkaline in order to function properly. The foods recommended on Atkins, however, are only acidic and neglect to bring balance to your body's pH. The health risks of failing to eat alkalizing foods, like the Super Carbs encouraged on the Fast Track program, can be disastrous because every system in the body was designed for an alkaline environment. Excessive acidity has also been strongly linked to bone loss by the National Institutes of Health.

— **Alcohol.** Alcohol is not approved on Atkins until after the induction phase, inviting those of us who want to relax with a glass of wine at night to cheat on the program almost immediately. On the Belly Fat Cure, you are allowed up to two glasses of alcohol like red wine (the ideal choice) each night. This ensures that even on Day 1, you feel encouraged rather than deprived.

— **Flora.** The final critical element that the Atkins diet neglects to correct is the problem that causes most low-carb dieters to fail: constipation. Most people have damaged or missing gut flora, which are absolutely vital to digestion, but treat only the symptoms of the problem with excessive fiber. Without repairing flora, the transition to an ideal lifestyle free of fiber supplements can be frustrating or downright impossible.

2. Do you still recommend the original *Belly Fat Cure* book?

Yes. The Belly Fat Cure program continues to work wonders because at its heart is the revolutionary concept that hidden sugars, not calories, cause weight gain. If you take only one thing away from any of my past or present books, it is that avoiding hidden sugar is the single most beneficial thing you can do for your weight loss and total health; for that reason, the original *Belly Fat Cure* is timeless.

Once you've discovered the new information and foods that the *Fast Track* edition has to offer, the first *Belly Fat Cure* book can serve several new purposes. Many of my Fast Track clients use it whenever they feel like going off the program temporarily, looking for satisfying products while still avoiding the biggest threat to their health: sugar.

Also, if you're looking for more great recipes, there are dozens of amazing meals that avoid hidden sugar in the original book. You can even quickly adapt most of the recipes from the original into Fast Track–approved options by performing the Ultimate Carb Swap. Simply swap the grains and starches of the original recipes for the Super Carbs of the Fast Track and you'll easily double your library of fat-melting recipes.

While I firmly believe that the Fast Track program can either help accelerate the results of the Belly Fat Cure or be used as a lifestyle all its own, the most important thing is that you pick a program that works for *your* lifestyle! Whichever strategy for defeating hidden sugar works best for you is absolutely the one you should stick with, because the benefits you experience from implementing any of the *Belly Fat Cure* books will transform your life.

3. Can my kids or grandkids eat in this way?

The answer is yes, absolutely! Removing sugar and grains from the diet and replacing them with vegetables and natural fats works just as well for those little ones who want to grow big and strong. All the same factors that make these foods excellent for the human body apply to kids and grandkids as well. The only trouble you may experience is changing their habits, but with a little creativity and commitment you can absolutely do it. Here's how!

— **Lead by example.** I recommend implementing the program in your own life before you set about trying to change the habits of your next generation. Just like an oxygen mask on an airplane, it's best to "secure your own" before you divert your attention to trying to change the attitudes of others. The better the results you experience yourself, and the better your mastery of the Fast Track foods and principles, the more powerful your influence will become.

— **Get them involved.** If they're under the age of five, simply prepare the same food for them that you would for yourself. There are no special foods or products that kids need, and again, their bodies prefer the same nutrients and energy that yours do. The only difference is that they are extremely impressionable in terms of the habits they learn from you at this age, regardless of their weight. Just because the 20 grams of sugar in that juice box won't make them fat overnight doesn't mean that it won't form bad habits that will cause them to be overweight and unhealthy in the near future . . . or as adults.

Just like that critical window in a young person's life where they're able to pick up other languages with ease, this is the window where your kids can learn healthy habits that will preserve their health for a lifetime. It is the habits you pass on, not your genes, that will have the greatest impact on their weight and health.

If they're older than five, I recommend waiting for them to ask about the changes you're making. Focus on improving your own health, weight, and choices and let your example spark their interest. All children are different, but pressuring them to eat in a certain way might not produce the desired effect.

Other ways in which you can get children over five involved is by educating them on the benefits of certain foods. I find that my kids are much more enthusiastic about eating foods like eggs and broccoli when they know that it will make them big and strong. Also, if they're a tad older than five, let them help you cook your meals. They will be much more inclined to take an interest in the food they eat if they also helped you create it.

— **Make it fun.** When it comes to kids of any age, it's all about the presentation. Sometimes the only thing a healthy food is missing is a miniature parasol or a brightly colored plastic sandwich sword. Try cookie cutters to form the foods I recommend in this program into different fun shapes. Or as I mentioned before, getting an older child involved in meal preparation will make the whole process of eating more fun. You just have to use a little extra creativity to get results for the whole family . . . kids and grandkids included!

For more tips on how to build healthier habits in your youngsters, check out an amazing joint venture between the Alliance for a Healthier Generation and the Michael & Susan Dell Foundation called Be Well. They offer free resources full of ideas from real parents at **BeWellBook.org**, or a paperback version may be ordered for less than $3 from **Amazon.com**.

4. I'm a vegetarian/vegan . . . can I do this program?

Yes, because anyone can do this program. While I still believe that animals are the most preferred source of protein, you can simply substitute the meats and/or cheeses I recommend in this program for your own favorite vegan or vegetarian options. I've also provided several more vegetarian/vegan-friendly options in a special section of the Belly Best Foods list on page 160.

If you do decide to use meat substitutes, just make sure that you know the sugar and carbohydrate content. One potential pitfall of the vegetarian lifestyle is that the predominant source of energy becomes carbohydrates rather than fats, which completely contradicts what makes this program work. So long as you eat the appropriate fats that come from nonanimal sources (or at least sources you feel are appropriate) like avocados, olive oil, and, nuts, you will achieve the hormonal balance that is the key to success on the Belly Fat Cure.

5. Do I really need to buy probiotics?

If you want to ensure a smooth transition to this lifestyle, I recommend beginning the program with probiotics. However, they may not be essential for you. Perhaps you haven't been exposed to the antibiotics and food additives that cause damage to your essential flora. You may certainly begin the program without taking probiotics, but if at some point you fail to have a bowel movement for 48 hours, then you should begin taking probiotics, and eat more Super Carbs immediately. Remember, constipation is the number one reason people fail on generally low-carb or grain-free diets.

6. So are all the Belly Good foods you recommended in the original *Belly Fat Cure* book, like Ezekiel 4:9 bread, really full of sugar?

No. The Belly Good foods and products I recommended in the original *Belly Fat Cure* book are still much better than most conventional products in their categories. If you're going to have a piece of toast, I'd still recommend you use bread that is low in, or free of, simple sugars. However, if you want to lose weight faster with the BFC Fast Track program, I highly recommend that you obtain your carbs from the most ideal sources, such as vegetables.

Using the products I recommend in the first book works because they limit insulin production. The recommendations in this book simply work *faster* because *insulin is even lower and glucagon even higher.* Although I say throughout the book that grains and starches are sugar in disguise, they aren't literally the simple carbohydrates that we think of as sugar. However, all carbohydrates eventually stimulate insulin, which is exactly why this program only recommends carbohydrates from the most nutrient-dense sources.

7. I'm taking probiotics, but things still aren't moving! What do I do?

It can take up to three months to fully restore your flora if it has been significantly damaged by antibiotics or artificial sweeteners like sucralose. I recommend patience as you regrow this lost "organ," but there are some steps you can take to get you through. The first is to eat more vegetables—I recommend broccoli and artichokes for their ideal fiber content—while you wait for your flora to regrow. If things are still sluggish after probiotics and ample Super Carbs, I recommend one or two servings of a soluble fiber supplement (see page 56 for my Digestion Perfection Checklist).

If patience, probiotics, extra Super Carbs, and one or two servings of a soluble fiber supplement still don't get things moving, there is one more solution. When you reduce the amount of carbohydrates in your diet, your body can go through a period of change. For most this is an automatic and unnoticeable process. But for some, the body begins to excrete or release sodium and potassium when on a low- or reduced-carbohydrate diet. Basically your kidneys start working overtime and start pulling sodium and storing water. Where are they going to get these materials? Your body pulls water from your bowels, making it difficult to have a bowel movement and bloating your body with excess water. Thus, while you are losing fat, your body is holding on to water and waste.

A simple solution is to replenish your sodium and potassium by drinking 16 ounces of chicken broth daily. This will regulate your body's chemical balance, and you can have a smooth bowel movement and avoid feeling fatigued.

8. How often should I weigh in?

In an ideal world, I'd be able to convince you to throw away your scale and judge your success on how you look and feel. If you do want to continue weighing yourself, however, make sure that you (1) use the same scale for each weigh-in; (2) place the scale on a hard floor rather than carpet; and (3) weigh yourself in the morning, preferably after a bowel movement. Always remember that your weight represents a combination of many different variables and shouldn't be obsessed about! I often find that my clients get discouraged by their scale, and discouragement impedes weight loss, so please be cautious about placing too much importance on your numerical weight.

9. Can I follow most of what is being said and still have a few carbs?

You *will* be eating carbs on this program. I merely recommend those that come with large doses of nutrients and are free of potentially inflammatory proteins . . . exactly the qualifications that make them Super Carbs (pages 159–160). That said, you are always free to eat whatever you like. My only goal is to provide you with the knowledge of which foods create health and which ones create hormonal havoc; the subsequent choices you make are up to you!

10. How long can I follow the Belly Fat Cure Fast Track program?

The Fast Track program can act as an accelerator to the original Belly Fat Cure program, or it can be followed indefinitely. In fact, there are only positive effects for sticking closely to the list of Belly Best Foods for as long as you like.

11. Can my parents or grandparents do this program?

Absolutely! There is not one recommendation in this book that wouldn't be ideal for older adults. Be advised that when someone is advanced in age, they may experience greater difficulty in correcting their digestion. For that reason, I recommend that anyone 65 or over absolutely begin the program with a probiotic supplement, plenty of Super Carbs, and two servings of a soluble fiber supplement.

12. What if I have a medical condition?

Always check with your doctor before starting any new eating program. However, keep in mind that not all medical professionals are dialed in to the changes in thinking (especially about fat and heart disease) that have emerged in the last few years. It may help to look up some of the studies listed in the Bibliography, and then bring printouts to discuss with your own physician.

13. You've created different diet books before that sometimes make different recommendations—did you make a mistake with your other books?

My other books were not mistakes, but rather represent my personal growth as a diet and fitness coach. My career began ten years ago, and I have acquired a wealth of new knowledge and new perspectives during that time.

14. Did I fail if I didn't lose 14 pounds in 14 days?

Absolutely not! No matter how much weight you lost, if you followed my instructions, then your body is eternally grateful for what you've done for it. If you're disappointed in your numerical results, simply ask yourself, "How do I feel?" I've never had a Fast Track client fail to express a complete change in his or her energy level, mood, and confidence. Keep in mind that weight loss depends on many factors, and you should never give up on yourself or your goals.

15. Where do I submit my story?

I want to hear all about your success! Share your story, along with before-and-after photos, on my Facebook page: **Facebook.com/JorgeCruise**

16. Won't the cholesterol in things like butter and egg yolks cause heart disease and death? And if the food I'm eating is high in cholesterol, won't my cholesterol levels go up?

These are common questions from my clients, as we've been conditioned to believe that saturated fat will kill us by causing heart disease. We are fortunate to live in a time when numerous studies are refuting this misconception, finding no link between dietary cholesterol and dangerous levels of LDL or triglycerides.

17. You don't seem to set any limits with respect to proteins, fats, and veggies. Can I eat too much?

You can eat too much of anything. If you take my recommendations on assessing your hunger (page 86) or follow my strategies for overcoming compulsive eating (Chapter 7), you can avoid eating too much food . . . as well as avoiding the regret that soon follows.

18. Am I ever going to eat fruit again?

While fruit may sometimes be problematic for weight loss because of its sugar content, I make recommendations for how to incorporate the best fruits into this edition of the Belly Fat Cure on page 161.

19. Will I feel awful the first week? Is there an induction phase?

There is no induction phase, because the goal of this program isn't ketosis, but rather, optimal health. Depending on your prior levels of sugar intake, however, you may experience some symptoms of withdrawal. They typically last no longer than a week, and I recommend combatting any resulting sugar cravings by always satiating hunger with good fats and Restorative Proteins.

20. How will I get enough energy?

Your new energy source will be the good fats you consume, as well as the energy from tapping into your stored body fat.

21. What is a safe amount of weight loss per week?

While "weight" loss per week can vary dramatically as a result of several different factors, a safe amount of pure fat loss per week is around two to three pounds of fat, depending on how much you have to lose. (See page 4 for more information.)

22. Can I still run marathons and do this program?

A common misconception is that runners or endurance athletes need lots of complex carbs for energy. However, even runners and endurance athletes will do their bodies a favor by switching to a fat-burning metabolism instead of a carb-burning (and fat-storing) metabolism. Our ancestors needed plenty of energy for endurance, yet for 99 percent of our time on Earth, they had no access to what *we* think of as carbs (breads, pastas, and so on). My favorite snack for endurance athletes is a big handful of macadamia nuts, which provide the ideal balance of good fats for sustained energy.

23. Can I work out and do this program?

Absolutely, so long as you understand the importance of balancing your workouts with adequate rest (page 186).

24. Can I ever have grains again?

You are always permitted to eat whatever you want. My goal in this book is simply to dispel the myths surrounding grains, and allow you to make as informed a decision as possible.

25. What do I do if I'm still hungry at the end of the day?

I recommend a snack, good fat, or Restorative Protein. If this doesn't satisfy your hunger, please re-read Chapter 7.

26. What should I do if I'm not losing weight?

Something that is stimulating insulin may be hidden in your food, and I recommend checking all dressings, sauces, and drinks for sugar or artificial sweeteners. You may also benefit from employing the strategies I recommend on pages 90–91.

27. Do I have to drink 8 to 10 glasses of water each day?

Not necessarily. I recommend using your thirst and the appearance of your urine as a guide to determine your own personal levels of adequate hydration. (See page 88 for more information.)

28. Can I drink as much coffee or tea as I want to in a day?

I recommend drinking no more than two cups of coffee throughout the day, as you run the risk of becoming dependent on caffeine. For optimal health and energy, I encourage you to try switching to green tea, which you are allowed in essentially unlimited amounts. A squeeze of lemon in your green tea boosts its health and anticancer benefits immensely.

29. What are good fats?

These are natural and not derived from a chemical or industrial process. They include animal fats, olive oil, coconut oil, avocados, butter, and cream. For a more complete list, see pages 158–159.

FAST TRACK
SUCCESS
STORY

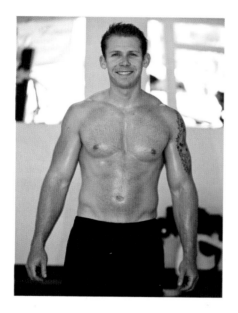

Before

Age: 25
Height: 5'7"
Pounds Lost: 9

Before meeting Jorge and discovering the innovations at the heart of the Fast Track program, I was in pretty good shape and thought I already knew everything I needed. After studying fitness and nutrition in college, I put the conventional wisdom I'd learned into practice and believed that there weren't any real alternatives. As I said, I looked and felt pretty good but could never seem to break through the plateau that kept me from reaching my highest potential.

As a personal trainer and wellness educator, I work with hundreds of clients in a gym setting and have the potential to work myself out endlessly . . . all day, every day if I chose to! But that only got me so far, and seemed to create a subconscious excuse to eat whatever I wanted.

Then I met Jorge, and he put forth an idea that a lot of guys have a hard time believing at first: the way your body looks is determined 90 percent by diet and 10 percent by exercise. When I first started the Fast Track, I weighed 162 pounds and had 8 percent body fat. Not too shabby, right? But after just 14 days of implementing Jorge's recommendations, which included many delicious foods I'd always been told to avoid, I lost 9 pounds and dropped to a truly shredded 5 percent body fat! I've never been this lean or felt this great in my life. After seeing such a rapid transformation, and all without altering my fitness regimen, my fellow trainers are jealous, and my clients are more motivated than ever . . . the perfect combination.

Stephen
Lost 9 pounds!

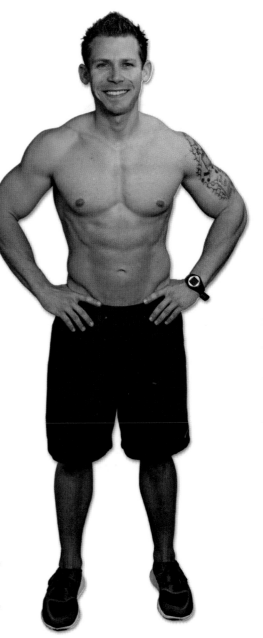

What's Next?

These days I educate my clients about the health benefits of switching to good fats for energy and Super Carbs for fiber and other nutrients, in addition to exercise. I've had multiple clients lose up to 12 pounds in two weeks while also feeling more energetic.

My Best Tip

For those of us who consider ourselves fit and healthy already, it can be extremely difficult to release certain aspects of conventional wisdom. It is critical that you open your mind to new ideas and break old habits in order to discover what your body may be missing.

Also, I eat lots of raw nuts as snacks to keep me going when I have a number of clients back to back. One night a week I roast a bunch of them myself, either on the stovetop or on a baking sheet in the oven, to enhance their flavor and make them more enjoyable. Having them on hand wherever I go has been critical to making the right choices every day.

FAST TRACK
SUCCESS
STORY

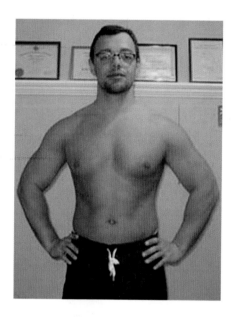

Before

Age: 34
Height: 5'6"
Pounds Lost: 17

Like a lot of people, my path to getting in better shape started with noticing myself in the mirror one day. I realized that even though I was working out five or six times every week, I seemed to be gaining weight. For all the time and effort I was spending at the gym, I still thought I looked fat and was definitely headed in the wrong direction.

I decided to give the "low-carb lifestyle" a shot, even though I'd heard a lot of mixed opinions about it. I stopped counting calories, even though my friends advised against it. Instead, I started paying closer attention to sugar and carbohydrates on every food label, and really any food that I would eat.

It wasn't long until the change in my diet delivered that elusive six-pack, which for men is like the gold medal of fitness and confidence. My workout routine hadn't changed at all . . . it was the food I was eating that had been holding me back all along. On top of the improvements in my appearance and confidence, my energy is better than ever, and I attribute that change to the fact that I get my energy from good fats like eggs, avocados, and olive oil.

I went to Jorge's Facebook page and posted my before-and-after photos, and within a few days I received an e-mail from Jorge about being in his newest book. It was crazy! I'm so glad I shared the success I experienced on the program because now I'm more motivated than ever, and it's a great feeling to think that someone else may see my photos and realize that they can do it, too!

Robert
Lost 17 pounds!

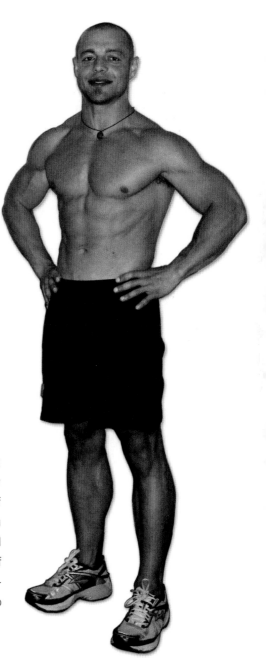

What's Next?

I love fitness, so I'm still very active and hit the gym often. Now I enjoy it even more because I have more energy to put into it. I'm now training for my third marathon and am excited to train for my first-ever triathlon, something I wouldn't have dreamed of doing with my old body and energy level. I've set a long-term goal for myself of qualifying for the Boston Marathon, and the thought of such an achievement really keeps me motivated!

My Best Tip

Find an activity that you enjoy and work it into your schedule. I'm lucky that I actually enjoy being at the gym. Also, I'm a big fan of what some people call the 90/10 principle. You just need to remember that you're human, and your nutrition won't be perfect 100 percent of the time. Recognize that fact, shoot for 90 percent of the time, and don't beat yourself up about it!

Fast Track Menu
Shopping Lists

SHOPPING LIST: WEEK 1

PROTEINS
Bacon
Chicken breast
Deli meat (select
  your favorites)
Eggs
Ground chuck
Halibut
Pork chops
Salmon
Steak (any cut)
Tilapia
Tuna

**SUPER CARBS
(VEGETABLES)**
Artichokes
Asparagus
Broccoli
Cauliflower
Cucumbers
Lettuce
Mixed greens

Mushrooms
Peppers (select
  your favorites)
Spinach

SNACKS
Almonds
Cheese (string
  or waxed is
  recommended)
Cottage cheese
Macadamia nuts
Pecans
Pumpkin seeds
Walnuts

SKINNY FATS
Avocado
Butter
Cheese (select
  your favorites)
Olive oil-and-
  vinegar dressing

TREATS
Club soda (as
  desired)
Cocoa powder
  (unsweetened)
Dark chocolate
  (85%)
Red wine (as
  desired)
Vodka (as desired)
Whipped cream
  (1 gram of sugar
  or less per
  serving)

SEASONINGS
Cinnamon
Pepper
Salt

OTHER
Coffee
Half-and-half

SHOPPING LIST: WEEK 2

PROTEINS
Bacon
Chicken breast
Deli meat (select
  your favorites)
Eggs
Ground beef
Halibut
Pork chops
Salmon
Sausage
Steak (any cut)
Tilapia
Tuna

**SUPER CARBS
(VEGETABLES)**
Artichokes
Asparagus
Broccoli
Cauliflower
Cucumbers
Lettuce
Mixed greens
Mushrooms
Peppers (select
  your favorites)
Spinach

Squash
Zucchini

SNACKS
Almonds
Brazil nuts
Cheese (string
  or waxed is
  recommended)
Cottage cheese
Macadamia nuts
Pumpkin seeds
Sunflower seeds
Walnuts

SKINNY FATS
Avocado
Butter
Cheese (select your
  favorites)
Olive oil-and-vinegar
  dressing

TREATS
Club soda (as desired)
Cocoa powder
  (unsweetened)
Dark chocolate (85%)

Red wine (as desired)
Vodka (as desired)
Whipped cream
  (1 gram of sugar
  or less per serving)

SEASONINGS
Cinnamon
Pepper
Salt

OTHER
Coffee
Half-and-half

Costco, Target, Walmart, and Sam's Club
Grocery Food Lists

For those of you who like to do your grocery shopping at Costco, Target, Walmart, or Sam's Club, here are lists of Fast Track–approved items that can be found in each store.

Costco Shopping List

Kirkland Signature:

Albacore tuna

Artichoke hearts marinated in oil

Atlantic salmon

Atlantic salmon, canned

Boneless skinless chicken breast

Boneless skinless chicken tenderloins

California pistachios

Cashew nuts

Chicken breast, canned in water

Chunk chicken breast, canned

Classic roast beef top round

Cooked salad shrimp

Crumbled bacon

Diet green tea with citrus

Dry-roasted almonds

Dry-roasted & salted almonds

Extra fancy mixed nuts

Fancy shredded Mexican
    4-cheese blend

Frozen shrimp

Fully cooked bacon

Grilled chicken breast strips

Ground sirloin burger

Halved pecans

Japanese green tea

Lean ground beef

Low-moisture part-skim
    mozzarella cheese

Low-sodium bacon

Natural shredded cheddar Jack cheese

Oven-roasted deli-sliced turkey breast

Parmigiano-Reggiano cheese

Parmigiano-Reggiano cheese, shredded

Premium chunk chicken breast

Raw tail-on shrimp

Roast beef, canned

Sirloin beef patties

Sliced bacon

Smoked Black Forest ham

Solid white albacore tuna

Turkey burgers

Wild Alaskan sockeye salmon, canned

Wild Pacific mahi mahi

Target Shopping List

Archer Farms:

Bacon-wrapped chicken breast fillets

Garlic & herb chicken breast skewers

Mahi mahi fillets

Raw almonds

Roasted almonds, salted

Market Pantry:

Boneless skinless chicken breast

Cheddar Jack cheese, finely shredded

Chicken breast in water

Chunk light tuna in water

Colby Jack cheese snack sticks

Colby Jack deli cheese slices

Cottage cheese, 4% milkfat

Deli Swiss cheese slices

Garlic herb boneless, skinless
    chicken breast

Grilled chicken strips fajita

Jamaican chicken wings

Lemon herb boneless, skinless
    chicken breast

Original beef stick

Parmesan cheese, 100% grated

Pepper Jack cheese snack bars

Tilapia fillets

Wild flounder fillets

Sutton & Dodge:

Angus beef steak

Beef chunk tender steak

Beef cubed steak

Beef eye of round steak

Beef top round steak

Boneless beef prime rib roast

Boneless loin strip steak

Petite sirloin steak

Sirloin steak

Stew meat

Walmart and Sam's Club Shopping List

Great Value:

100% extra virgin olive oil

100% Parmesan grated cheese

100% pure individually quick-frozen
    beef patties

Alaskan pink salmon

All-natural sour cream

All-natural tea

Beef burgers

California ripe olives, chopped

California ripe olives, large pitted

California ripe olives, medium pitted

Chicken wing drummettes

Colby & Monterey Jack cheese

Colby & Monterey Jack cheese,
    shredded

Collard greens

Cooked ham

Cream of mushroom condensed soup

Dijon mustard

Dill pickle spears

Fiesta blend cheese, finely shredded

Luncheon meat

Medium cheddar cheese

Mild cheddar cheese

Mild cheddar cheese, fancy shredded

Mild, easy-to-open green chilies

Minced pimiento-stuffed
    manzanilla olives

Mustard greens

Natural Monterey Jack cheese

Orange smoked oysters

Pieces & stems canned mushrooms

Potted meat

Powdered garlic

Premium fully cooked chunk chicken

Premium ground coffee

Pure olive oil

Real bacon pieces

Real mayonnaise

Sauerkraut

Sharp cheddar cheese

Soy sauce

Vienna sausage

Whole jalapeños

Whole leaf spinach

Worcestershire sauce

Optional
Specialty Brands

These products can be found at **TheBellyFatCure.com** or at your local health-food store, and can be a part of your Fast Track lifestyle because they use smart and natural sweeteners:

Sweeteners

Pure Via
SweetLeaf Sweetener
Truvia
XyloSweet

Barlean's Organic Oils

Coconut oil
The Essential Woman Swirl,
     chocolate raspberry
Flax oil, cinnamon
Flax oil, lemonade

Kid's Omega Swirl, lemonade
Olive Leaf Complex
Omega Man
Omega Swirl, blackberry
Omega Swirl, lemon zest
Omega Swirl, mango peach
Omega Swirl, piña colada
Omega Swirl, strawberry
     banana
Total Omega Swirl, orange
     cream
Total Omega Vegan Swirl,
     pomegranate blueberry

Nature's Hollow

Sugar-free BBQ sauce, hickory maple
Sugar-free BBQ sauce, honey mustard
Sugar-free honey
Sugar-free jam, apricot
Sugar-free jam, mountain berry
Sugar-free jam, peach
Sugar-free jam, raspberry
Sugar-free jam, strawberry
Sugar-free jam, wild blueberry
Sugar-free ketchup
Sugar-free syrup, maple
Sugar-free syrup, raspberry

Steaz

Zero Calorie Sparkling Green Tea
    Black cherry
    Blueberry pomegranate
    Orange
    Raspberry

Xlear, Inc.

SparX candies, berry
SparX candies, citrus
SparX candies, fruit

Spry gum, cinnamon
Spry gum, fresh fruit
Spry gum, green tea
Spry gum, peppermint
Spry gum, spearmint
Spry mints, berryblast
Spry mints, lemonburst
Spry mints, power peppermints

Zevia

All Natural Soda
    Black Cherry
    Caffeine Free Cola
    Cola
    Cream Soda
    Dr. Zevia
    Ginger Ale
    Ginger Root Beer
    Grape
    Grapefruit Citrus
    Lemon Lime Twist
    Mountain Zevia
    Orange

Index of
Recipes

Beef & Pork Dishes

Egg Dishes

Fish & Seafood Dishes

Meatless Dishes

Poultry

Salads

Sauces and Dips

Smart Carbs

Belly Fat Cure Cheesy Parmesan Crisps (page 103)
Belly Fat Cure Sweet Chocolate Mousse Crêpes (page 95)
Ryan's Portobello Mini-Pizzas (page 143)
Sweet Ricotta Pancakes (page 123)
Zucchini Cheese Fries (page 147)

Treats

Belly Fat Cure Sweet Chocolate Mousse Crêpes (page 95)
Jorge's Chocolate Lace Cookies (page 113)
Itty Bitty Nutty Pie (page 153)
Macadamia Nut Clusters (page 149)
Sweet Surprise Cottage Cheese (page 151)

Glossary

Alkalizing: Foods that bring balance to your body's pH by causing your system to become more alkaline after digestion. Plants like Super Carbs are your body's ideal alkalizing foods. (Page 35)

Autoimmune disorders: Disorders that arise from the immune system attacking normal cells in the body. Common autoimmune disorders include arthritis, psoriasis, narcolepsy, lupus, multiple sclerosis, and perhaps even schizophrenia and Alzheimer's. Many now believe the underlying cause of these diseases is incorrect diet. (Page 37)

Belly Best Foods: The Fast Track foods that keep glucagon levels exceptionally high by keeping insulin low. (Page 88)

Calcium balance: Not just how much calcium you consume, but how much you absorb and how much you retain. Healthy calcium balance is aided by vitamin D, magnesium, and alkalizing foods. (Page 35)

Calorie myth, The: Often referred to as "calories in, calories out," this myth assumes that calorie intake is the only factor involved in successful weight control. (Page 10)

Celiac disease: On the most grain-intolerant end of the spectrum, those with celiac disease have a genetically linked and potentially life-threatening autoimmune response to gluten. (Page 36)

Compelling future: A positive event that could occur in the future if you make the right choices. This event or outcome should be so attractive that it is a powerful motivator to make the right choices as often as you can. (Page 175)

Complex carbohydrates: Although these are absorbed more slowly, even complex carbs will eventually become simple carbs and drive the production of insulin. All carbs will cut in line as a fuel source, ensuring that the body never taps into stored fat . . . exactly why weight loss is accelerated when carbs come from only the most ideal sources. (Page 29)

Dickens diary: A journal in which you list the negative consequences that have occurred, continue to occur, or could occur as a result of making the wrong choices or continuing unhealthy habits. (Page 176)

Dietary fiber: Any soluble and insoluble fiber that accompanies the food we eat, with the most ideal sources being vegetables. (Page 48)

Dysbacteriosis: A condition widely overlooked in the West in which the gut loses its bacterial microflora, becoming sterile and unable to function as intended. Common disorders that result from dysbacteriosis include constipation and suppressed immune function. A deficiency in vitamin K, which is secreted by healthy flora, has also been linked to osteoporosis and coronary heart disease. (Page 49)

Endorphins: The body's mechanism for feeling blissful, this compound binds to receptor sites in the brain and induces a natural sense of well-being. (Page 31)

Energy: The power that we obtain from food and convert into movement, functions, and thoughts. (Page 89)

Energy deficit: A state of expending more energy than you consume. Only after hormonal balance has been achieved and a fat-burning metabolism has been created does encouraging an energy deficit become a helpful weight-loss tool. Focusing purely on the energy deficit—as Conventional Wisdom, Inc., suggests—leads to dieting, failure, and hunger. (Page 90)

False belly fat: Trapped waste matter that adds pounds and inches to the belly, and can also interfere with the absorption of nutrients and healthy digestion. (Page 6)

Farm Bill: The primary agricultural and food-policy tool of the federal government, in which billions of dollars are given to farmers as subsidies. The majority of the subsidies go toward some of the least ideal foods: corn, wheat, soybeans, and rice. (Page 39)

Fast Track Menu: The simplest and most delicious menu of nutritious foods that keep your belly fat loss at the maximum. (Page 65)

Fiber myth, The: The belief that essential dietary fiber and "high-fiber food products" made from grains are the same thing. (Page 47)

Fruit: Otherwise known as "nature's candy," it is the most nutritious and natural sweet treat out there. However, large amounts are not ideal for weight loss because of the sugar content. (Page 161)

Glucagon: The body's mechanism for shrinking fat tissue, this hormone is only capable of unlocking energy from fat cells when insulin is low. (Page 39)

Gluten: A composite protein found in some grass-related grains, most notably wheat, rye, and barley. While celiac disease is the most noticeable adverse reaction to gluten, it may also be the culprit for autoimmune responses in the larger segments of the general population sometimes referred to as "silent celiac." (Page 36)

Gut flora: The collection of microorganisms living in the human gut with which our bodies have evolved a symbiotic relationship. It is estimated that there are about 500 species living in the human body, and they perform metabolic activities that many compare to that of an organ. (Page 49)

Healthy goal weight: A weight and body composition at which you're both comfortable in your clothes and optimally healthy. Because of the body images we're exposed to daily, many people mistake a healthy goal weight for being "fat." (Page 89)

Hidden sugar: The sugar you consume without realizing it, or because you have been led to believe it is healthy. Classic examples include milk, fruit, yogurt, bread, juice, and practically every low-calorie or low-fat diet food ever created. (Page 1)

High-intensity interval training: The most effective cardio strategy for weight loss, the alternating intervals of medium to high intensity allow for the greatest energy to be spent in the shortest period of time. (Page 185)

Hygiene hypothesis: A recently popularized hypothesis that states a lack of exposure to infectious agents, symbiotic microorganisms, and parasites increases susceptibility to allergic diseases by hampering immune-system development. (Page 53)

Ideal: An option that is most beneficial to your weight loss and overall health, but not essential if it is unavailable or unaffordable. (Page 87)

Insulin: The regulator of blood sugar, this hormone also drives cells to burn carbohydrates instead of fat and indirectly stimulates the production of more fat. The imbalance of this critical hormone sets off a chain reaction that negatively impacts almost every corner of the body, and is the most profound health crisis facing our modern society. (Page 2)

Lectin: A protein found in foods like grains and legumes (beans) that recent studies have suggested may cause damage to the digestive system and resistance to the hormone leptin, which is a key hormone that regulates metabolism. Leptin resistance may lead to obesity in some. (Page 37)

Low-carb diet: A broad term that encompasses many diets that focus on reducing both simple and complex carbohydrates in order to lose weight. (Page 48)

Opioids: Any external substance that numbs pain and creates a feeling of euphoria, typically by mimicking the body's endorphins and often leading to dependence. (Page 31)

Paleolithic diet: A diet based on the nutrition available to the human species more than 10,000 years ago. This diet restricts foods that only became available due to modern agricultural and industrial processes. (Page 33)

Play: Movement and activity that increases your happiness and energy deficit without feeling like a chore or causing stress to the body. (Page 91)

Probiotics: Supplements that restore your gut flora and healthy digestion by delivering microorganisms to the intestines. If your flora is damaged or missing, these supplements are essential for restoring balance to your body and for losing weight. (Page 54)

Restorative Proteins: Natural protein from animals and plants that repairs and replaces damaged tissue in your body. (Page 87)

Simple carbohydrates: Most commonly referred to as sugar and quickly absorbed into the bloodstream, simple carbohydrates drive the production of insulin and feed the blood-sugar roller coaster. (Page 29)

Snack: A source of energy and nutrients that is designed to get you safely from one meal to the next, without falling victim to some food that will reverse your weight loss. (Page 87)

Super Carbs: Low-sugar vegetables that provide you with the ideal source of carbohydrates and dietary fiber while also providing balance to your body's pH. (Page 32)

Supplemental fiber: Soluble or insoluble fiber that is added to the diet as a means of promoting healthy digestion. While also part of a healthy lifestyle, this may not correct the underlying cause of irregularity or poor digestion. (Page 50)

Symbiotic: A relationship between two organisms in which one or both benefit from the functions of the other. (Page 50)

Treats: Foods that will not directly help you lose weight, but may keep you sane and on course while satisfying your sweet tooth. (Page 87)

Ujjayi: An ancient breathing technique that helps quiet the mind and bring one's focus to the breath. Deep breathing such as Ujjayi is the body's "emotional digestive system." (Page 170)

Ultimate Carb Swap: Exchanging carbs from sugar, starches, and grains for the nutrient-dense Super Carbs. (Page 30)

Bibliography

Chapter 1: 14 Pounds in 14 Days

Chaput, Jean-Philippe, et al. "A Novel Interaction Between Dietary Composition and Insulin Secretion: Effects on Weight Gain in the Quebec Family Study." *The American Journal of Clinical Nutrition* 87.2 (2008): 303–309.

Crowley, Leonard V. "The Pancreas and Diabetes Mellitus." An *Introduction to Human Disease: Pathology and Pathophysiology Correlations.* Sudbury: Jones & Bartlett Learning, 2004. 589–605.

Ebbeling, Cara B., et al. "Effects of a Low-Glycemic Load vs. Low-Fat Diet in Obese Young Adults." *The Journal of the American Medical Association* 297.19 (2007): 2092–2102.

Mattes, R. D., and D. Donnelly. "Relative contributions of dietary sodium sources." *Journal of the American College of Nutrition* 10.4 (1991): 383–393.

Moyer, Melinda Wenner. "Carbs Against Cardio: More Evidence that Refined Carbohydrates, not Fats, Threaten the Heart." Scientific American May 2010: 19–21.

Oliver, J. Eric. *Fat Politics: The Real Story Behind America's Obesity Epidemic.* Oxford: Oxford University Press, 2006.

Rasheed, Al Assad. "Carbohydrate Intake, Inflammation and the Metabolic Syndrome." Al Assad Rasheed, Ph.D.'s blog on Talk Medical. http://talk.news-medical.net/profiles/blogs/carbohydrate-intake.

Samaha, Frederick F., et al. "A Low-Carbohydrate as Compared with a Low-Fat Diet in Severe Obesity." *The New England Journal of Medicine* 348.21 (2003): 2074–2081.

Shai, Iris, et al. "Weight Loss with a Low-Carbohydrate, Mediterranean, or Low-Fat Diet." *The New England Journal of Medicine* 359.3 (2008): 229–241.

Sherrid, Pamela. "Piling on the Profit: There's No Slimming Down for Companies Selling Diet Products." *US News & World Report* 16 Mar. 2003: 41–43.

Taubes, Gary. "What if It's All Been a Big Fat Lie?" *The New York Times Magazine* 7 July 2002: 22–27.

United States Department of Defense. "Fiscal Year 2011 Budget Request." http://comptroller .defense.gov/budget.html.

United States Department of Health & Human Services. "Fiscal Year 2010 Buget in Brief: Centers for Medicare & Medicaid Services." http://dhhs.gov/asfr/ob /docbudget/2010budgetinbriefk.html.

United States Department of the Treasury Bureau of the Public Debt. "Interest Expense on the Debt Outstanding." TreasuryDirect. http://www.treasurydirect.gov/govt/reports/ir/ ir_expense.htm.

Wang, Youfa, et al. "Will All Americans Become Overweight or Obese? Estimating the Progression and Cost of the US Obesity Epidemic." *Obesity* 16.10 (2008): 2323–2330.

Williams, Elizabeth M. "The Sixth Deadly Sin." *Gastronomica* 6.3 (2006): 60–3.

Yancy, William S., et al. "A Low-Carbohydrate, Ketogenic Diet versus a Low-Fat Diet to Treat Obesity and Hyperlipidemia." *Annals of Internal Medicine* 140.10 (2004): 769–777.

Chapter 2: The Ultimate Carb Swap

Akunne, H. C., and K. F. A. Soliman. "The role of opioid receptors in diabetes and hyper-glycemia-induced changes in pain threshold in the rat." *Psychopharmacology* 93.2 (1987): 167–172.

American Autoimmune Related Diseases Association, Inc. "Mission Statement." http://aarda .org/mission_statement.php.

Braly, James, and Ron Hoggan. Dangerous *Grains: Why Gluten Cereal Grains May Be Hazardous to Your Health.* New York: Avery, 2002.

Cohen, Sarah, Dan Morgan, and Laura Stanton. "Farm Subsidies Over Time." *The Washington Post.* 2 July 2006. http://washingtonpost.com/wpdyn/content/graphic/2006/07/02 /GR2006070200024.html.

Cordain, Loren. "Cereal grains: Humanity's double-edged sword." *World Review of Nutrition and Dietetics* 84 (1999): 19–73.

Cordain, Loren, Janette Brand Miller, S. Boyd Eaton, Neil Mann, Susanne Holt, and John Speth. "Plant-animal subsistence ratios and macro-nutrient energy estimations in worldwide hunter-gather diets." *The American Journal of Clinical Nutrition* 71 (2000): 682–692.

Cordain, Loren, L. Toohey, M.J. Smith, and M.S. Hickey. "Modulation of immune function by dietary lectins in rheumatoid arthritis." *British Journal of Nutrition* 83 (2000): 207–17.

Cordain, Loren, et al. "Origins and evolution of the Western diet: health implications for the 21st century." *The American Journal of Clinical Nutrition* 81.2 (2005): 341–354.

D'Andrea, Michael R. "Add Alzheimer's disease to the list of autoimmune diseases." *Medical Hypotheses* 64.3 (2005): 458–63.

Eaton, S. Boyd. "The ancestral human diet: what was it and should it be a paradigm for contemporary nutrition?" *Proceedings of the Nutrition Society* 65.1 (2006): 1–6.

Eaton, S. Boyd, and M. Konner. "Paleolithic nutrition: a consideration of its nature and current implications." *New England Journal of Medicine* 312 (1985): 283–289.

Eaton, William W., et al. "Association of schizophrenia and autoimmune diseases: linkage of Danish national registers." *The American Journal of Psychiatry* 163.3 (2006): 521–528.

Frassetto, L. A., et al. "Metabolic and physiologic improvements from consuming a Paleolithic, hunter-gatherer type diet." *European Journal of Clinical Nutrition* 63 (2009): 947–955.

Freed, David L. J. "Do dietary lectins cause disease?" *The British Journal of Medicine* 318 (1999): 1023–1024.

Jenkins, David J. A., et al. "Glycemic index: overview of implications in health and disease." *American Journal of Clinical Nutrition* 76.S1 (2002): 266–273.

Johnson, Richard J., et al. "Potential role of sugar (fructose) in the epidemic of hypertension, obesity and the metabolic syndrome, diabetes, kidney disease, and cardiovascular disease." *American Journal of Clinical Nutrition* 86.4 (2007): 899–906.

Jones, Amanda L., et al. "Immune dysregulation and self-reactivity in schizophrenia: Do some cases of schizophrenia have an autoimmune basis?" *Immunology and Cell Biology* 83.1 (2005): 9–17.

Kather, H., and B. Simon. "Opioid peptides and obesity." *Lancet* 2 (1979): 905.

Lindeberg, S., et al. "A Palaeolithic diet improves glucose tolerance more than a Mediterranean-like diet in individuals with ischaemic heart disease." *Diabetologia* 50 (2007): 1795–1807.

Mercola, Joseph, and Alison Rose Levy. *The No-Grain Diet: Conquer Carbohydrate Addiction and Stay Slim for Life.* New York: Penguin, 2004.

National Digestive Diseases Information Clearinghouse. "Celiac Disease." National Institute of Diabetes and Digestive and Kidney Diseases, National Institutes of Health. http://digestive .niddk.nih.gov/ddiseases/pubs/celiac.

National Psoriasis Foundation. "About Psoriasis." http://psoriasis.org/netcommunity/learn/about-psoriasis.

Riedl, Brian. "Still at the Federal Trough: Farm Subsidies for the Rich and Famous Shattered Records in 2001." The Heritage Foundation. http://heritage.org/Research/Reports/2002/04/Farm-Subsidies-for-the-Rich-amp-Famous-Shattered-Records-in-2001.

Sisson, Mark. *The Primal Blueprint*. Malibu: Primal Nutrition, Inc., 2009.

Smith, Melissa Diane. *Going Against the Grain: How Reducing and Avoiding Grains Can Revitalize Your Health*. New York: McGraw-Hill, 2002.

Stattin, Pär, et al. "Prospective Study of Hyperglycemia and Cancer Risk." *Diabetes Care* 30.3 (2007): 561–567.

Strous, Rael D., and Yehuda Shoenfeld. "Schizophrenia, autoimmunity and immune system dysregulation: A comprehensive model updated and revisited." *Journal of Autoimmunity* 27.2 (2006): 71–80.

"United States Farm Bills." The National Agricultural Law Center. http://nationalaglawcenter.org/farmbills.

University of Chicago Celiac Disease Center. "Celiac Disease Facts and Figures." The University of Chicago Medical Center. http://uchospitals.edu/pdf/uch_007937.pdf.

Vogel, Stephen. "Farm Income and Costs: Farms Receiving Government Payments." United States Department of Agriculture, Economic Research Service. http://ers.usda.gov/briefing/farmincome/govtpaybyfarmtype.htm.

Wadley, G., and A. Martin. "The Origins of Agriculture: A Biological Perspective and a New Hypothesis." *Australian Biologist* 6 (1993): 96–105.

Zioudrou, C., R. A. Streaty, and W. A. Klee. "Opioid peptides derived from food proteins: The exorphins." *Biological Chemistry* 254 (1979): 2446–2449.

Chapter 3: Ensuring Your Success

Abdul-Hamid, Azizah, and Yu Siew Luan. "Functional properties of dietary fibre prepared from defatted rice bran." *Food Chemistry* 68.1 (2000): 15–19.

Chuan-Ke, Duan, Jiang Dao-Ping, and Wang Yu-Shen. "Dysbacteriosis caused by antibiotics, and its prevention and cure." *Chinese Pharmacological Bulletin* S1 (1998).

Cordain, Loren, L. Toohey, M.J. Smith, and M.S. Hickey. "Modulation of immune function by dietary lectins in rheumatoid arthritis." *British Journal of Nutrition* 83 (2000): 207–217.

Farhadi, Ashkan, et al. "Intestinal barrier: An interface between health and disease." *Journal of Gastroenterology and Hepatology* 18.5 (2003): 479–497.

Fleming, John O., and Thomas D. Cook. "Multiple sclerosis and the hygiene hypothesis." *Neurology* 67.11 (2006): 2085–2086.

Fooks, L. J., and G. R. Gibson. "Probiotics and modulators of the gut flora." *British Journal of Nutrition* 88 (2002): 39S–49S.

Furzikova, T. M., et al. "The effect of antibiotic preparations and their combinations with probiotics on the intestinal microflora of mice." *Mikrobiolohichnyi zhurnal* 62.3 (2000): 26–35.

Hill, M. J. "Intestinal flora and endogenous vitamin synthesis." *European Journal of Cancer Prevention* 6.2 (1997): S43–S45.

International Foundation for Functional Gastrointestinal Disorders. "Facts About IBS." http://aboutibs.org/site/about-ibs/facts-about-ibs.

Isolauri, Erika, et al. "Probiotics: effects on immunity." *American Journal of Clinical Nutrition* 73.2 (2001): 444S–450S.

Kaufman, Stefan. "Immunology's foundation: the 100-year anniversary of the Nobel Prize to Paul Ehrlich and Elie Metchnikoff." *Nature Immunology* 9 (2008): 705–712.

Kaufman, Wendy. "Atkins Bankruptcy a Boon for Pasta Makers." NPR. http://npr.org/templates/story/story.php?storyId=4783324.

Klauser, A. G., et al. "Behavioral modification of colonic function. Can constipation be learned?" *Digestive Diseases and Sciences* 35.10 (1990): 1271–1275.

Koloski, Natasha A., Laurel Bret, and Graham Radford-Smith. "Hygiene hypothesis in inflammatory bowel disease: A critical review of the literature." *World Journal of Gastroenterology* 14.2 (2008): 165–173.

Mariani, Giuliano, et al. "Radionuclide Evaluation of the Lower Gastrointestinal Tract." *Journal of Nuclear Medicine* 49.5 (2008): 776–787.

Mayo Clinic staff. "High-Fiber Foods." The Mayo Clinic. http://mayoclinic.com/health/high-fiber-foods/NU00582.

McDonald, Lyle. *The Ketogenic Diet: A Complete Guide for the Dieter and Practitioner.* Austin, TX: Lyle McDonald, 1998.

O'Hara, Ann M., and Fergus Shanahan. "The gut flora as a forgotten organ." *The European Molecular Biology Organization Reports* 7.7 (2006): 688–693.

Rubin, Jordan S., and Joseph Brasco. *Restoring Your Digestive Health: How the Guts and Glory Program Can Transform Your Life.* New York: Kensington Publishing Corp., 2003.

Schmidt, Robert, and Gerhard Thews. "Colonic Motility." *Human Physiology.* New York: Springer-Verlag, 1989.

Strachan, David P. "Hay fever, hygiene and household size." *British Medical Journal* 299 (1989): 1259–60.

Vander, Arthur J., James H. Sherman, and Dorothy S. Luciano. "The Digestion and Absorption of Food." *Human Physiology: The Mechanisms of Body Function.* Columbus: McGraw-Hill, 2001.

Wood, Heather. "Fiber Dietary Supplements." Livestrong.com. http://livestrong.com/article/84551-fiber-dietary-supplements.

Zaphiropoulos, G. C. "Rheumatoid arthritis and the gut." *British Journal of Rheumatology* 25.2 (1986): 138–140.

Zhou, QiQi, Buyi Zhang, and G. Nicholas Verne. "Intestinal membrane permeability and hypersensitivity in the irritable bowel syndrome." *Pain* 146.1 (2009): 41–46.

Chapter 4: The 14-Day Challenge and Beyond

Blundell, J. E., V. J. Burley, J. R. Cotton, and C. L. Lawton. "Dietary fat and the control of energy intake: evaluating the effects of fat on meal size and postmeal satiety." *American Journal of Clinical Nutrition* 57 (1993): 772–777.

Nestle, Marion. *Food Politics: How the Food Industry Influences Nutrition and Health.* Berkeley: University of California Press, 2007.

Ovaskainen, Marja-Leena. "Snacks as an element of energy intake and food consumption." *European Journal of Clinical Nutrition* 60 (2006): 494–501.

Rumessen, J. J. "Fructose and related food carbohydrates: sources, intake, absorption, and clinical implications." *Scandinavian Journal of Gastroenterology* 27.10 (1992): 819–28.

Schmidt, Robert F., and Gerhard Thews. "Water and Electrolyte Balance." *Human Physiology.* New York: Springer-Verlag, 1989.

Sisson, Mark. *The Primal Blueprint.* Malibu: Primal Nutrition, Inc., 2009.

Subcommittee on the Tenth Edition of the RDAs, Food and Nutrition Board, Commission on Life Sciences, National Research Council. *Recommended Dietary Allowances.* Washington, D.C.: National Academy Press, 1989.

Taubes, Gary. *Good Calories, Bad Calories: Challenging the Conventional Wisdom on Diet, Weight Control, and Disease.* New York: Alfred A. Knopf, 2007.

Valtin, Heinz. "'Drink at least eight glasses of water a day.' Really? Is there scientific evidence for '8 x 8'?" *American Journal of Physiology—Regulatory, Integrative, and Comparative Physiology* 283 (2002): 993–1004.

Chapter 7: Conquering an Addiction to Sugar

Hay, Louise. *You Can Heal Your Life.* Carlsbad, CA: Hay House, Inc., 1984.

Shapiro, Francine. "Eye movement desensitization: A new treatment for post-traumatic stress disorder." *Journal of Behavior Therapy and Experimental Psychiatry* 20.3 (1989): 211–217.

Shapiro, Francine, and Margot Silk Forrest. *EMDR: The Breakthrough "Eye Movement" Therapy for Overcoming Anxiety, Stress, and Trauma.* New York: Basic Books, 1997.

Chapter 8: Simply Fit™: Burn Belly Fat

Cloud, John. "Why Exercise Won't Make You Thin." *Time* 17 Aug. 2009: 42–47.

DeBusk, R. F., et al. "Training effects of long versus short bouts of exercise in healthy subjects." *The American Journal of Cardiology* 65.15 (1990): 1010–3.

Evans, William J., and Joseph G. Cannon. "The Metabolic Effects of Exercise-Induced Muscle Damage." *Exercise and Sport Sciences Reviews* 19.1 (1991): 99–126.

Lemon, Peter W. R. "Effects of Exercise on Protein Requirements." *Journal of Sports Sciences* 9.S1 (1991): 53–70.

McArdle, William D., Frank I. Katch, and Victor L. Katch. *Exercise Physiology: Energy, Nutrition, and Human Performance.* Philadelphia: Lippincott Williams & Wilkins, 2007.

National Center for Health Statistics. "Prevalence of overweight, obesity and extreme obesity among adults: United States, trends 1960–62 through 2005–2006." Centers for Disease Control and Prevention. http://cdc.gov/nchs/data/hestat/overweight/overweight_adult.htm.

Tipton, Charles M. *American College of Sports Medicine's Advanced Exercise Physiology.* Philadelphia: Lippincott Williams & Wilkins, 2006.

Tjonna, Arnt Erik, et al. "Aerobic Interval Training Versus Continuous Moderate Exercise as a Treatment for the Metabolic Syndrome: A Pilot Study." *Circulation* 118 (2008): 346–54.

Urhausen, A., H. Gabriel, and W. Kindermann. "Blood hormones as markers of training stress and overtraining." *Sports Medicine* 20.4 (1995), 251–76.

Verger, P., M. T. Lanteaume, and J. Louis-Sylvestre. "Human intake and choice of foods at intervals after exercise." *Appetite* 18.2 (1992): 93–99.

Warburton, Darren, Crystal Whitney Nicol, and Shannon Bredin. "Health benefits of physical activity: the evidence." *The Canadian Medical Association Journal* 174.6 (2006): 801–9.

Additional References

Attwood, Teresa K., and Richard Cammack. *Oxford Dictionary of Biochemistry and Molecular Biology.* Oxford: Oxford University Press, 2006.

Champe, Pamela C., Richard A. Harvey, and Denise R. Ferrier. "Metabolic Effects of Insulin and Glucagon." *Biochemistry.* Philadelphia: Lippincott Williams & Wilkins, 2005. 305–318.

Cheryan, Munir, and Joseph J. Rackis. "Phytic acid interactions in food systems." *Critical Reviews in Food Science and Nutrition* 13.4 (1980): 297–335.

Foster, Gary D., et al. "Weight and Metabolic Outcomes After 2 Years on a Low-Carbohydrate Versus Low-Fat Diet: A Randomized Trial." *Annals of Internal Medicine.* 153.3 (2010): 147–157.

Gardner, Christopher, Alexandre Kiazand, Sofiya Alhassan, Soowon Kim, Randall Stafford, Raymond Balise, Helena Kraemer, and Abby King. "Comparison of the Atkins, Zone, Ornish, and LEARN Diets for Change in Weight and Related Risk Factors Among Overweight Premenopausal Women." *Journal of The American Medical Association* 297.9 (2007): 969–977.

Gast, G. C. M., et al. "A high menaquinone intake reduces the incidence of coronary heart disease." *Nutrition, Metabolism, and Cardiovascular Disease* 19.7 (2009): 504–510.

Gibson, Glen R. "Fibre and effects on probiotics (the prebiotic concept)." *Clinical Nutrition Supplements* 1.2 (2004): 25–31.

Gilani G. Sarwar, Kevin A. Cockell, and Estatira Sepehr. "Effects of antinutritional factors on protein digestibility and amino acid availability in foods." *Journal of the Association of Official Analytical Chemists International* 88.3 (2005): 967–87.

Hallmayer, Joachim, et al. "Narcolepsy is strongly associated with the T-cell receptor alpha locus." *Nature Genetics* 41.5 (2009): 708–711.

Ikeda, Y., et al. "Intake of fermented soybeans, *natto,* is associated with reduced bone loss in postmenopausal women: Japanese population-based osteoporosis (JPOS) study." *Journal of Nutrition* 136.5 (2006): 1323–1328.

Jonsson, Tommy, Stefan Olsson, Bo Ahren, Thorkild C. Bog-Hansen, Anita Dole, and Staffan Lindeberg. "Agrarian diet and diseases of affluence—Do evolutionary novel dietary lectins cause leptin resistance?" *BioMed Central Endocrine Disorders* 5.10 (2005). http://biomed central.com/1472-6823/5/10.

Katsuyama, H., et al. "Usual dietary intake of fermented soybeans (natto) is associated with bone mineral density in premenopausal women." *Journal of Nutritional Science and Vitamin-ology* 48.3 (2002): 207–215.

Miyake, Katsuya, et al. "Lectin-based food poisoning: a new mechanism of protein toxicity." *PLoS ONE* 2.8 (2007). http://plosone.org/article/info:doi/10.1371/journal.pone.0000687.

Ogden, Cynthia L., Margaret Carroll, Margaret McDowell, and Katherine Flegal. "Obesity Among Adults in the United States—No Statistically Significant Change Since 2003–2004." NCHS Data Briefs, Centers for Disease Control and Prevention. http://cdc.gov/nchs/data/databriefs/db01.pdf.

Sano, M., et al. "Vitamin K$_2$ (menatetrenone) induces iNOS in bovine vascular smooth muscle cells: no relationship between nitric oxide production and gamma-carboxylation." *Journal of Nutritional Science and Vitaminology* 45.6 (1999): 711–723.

Schulman, Jerome L., et al. "Effect of Glucagon on Food Intake and Body Weight in Man." *Journal of Applied Physiology* 11 (1957): 419–21.

Sears, Cynthia L. "A dynamic partnership: Celebrating our gut flora." *Anaerobe* 11.5 (2005): 247–251.

Siri-Tarino, Patty, Qi Sun, Frank Hu, and Ronald Krauss. "Meta-analysis on prospective cohort studies evaluating the association of saturated fat with cardiovascular disease." *American Journal of Clinical Nutrition* 91.3 (2010): 535–546.

Steinhoff, Ulrich. "Who controls the crowd? New findings and old questions about the intestinal microflora." *Immunology Letters* 99.1 (2005): 12–16.

Strachan, David P. "Family size, infection and atopy: The first decade of the 'hygiene hypothesis.'" *Thorax* 55.S1 (2000): 2–10.

Willett, Walter C., and Rudolph L. Leibel. "Dietary fat is not a major determinant of body fat." *The American Journal of Medicine* 113.9S2 (2002): 47–59.

Acknowledgments

My deepest gratitude to Carol Brooks, Editor-in-Chief of *First for Women* magazine—it means so much that you share my mission of making a healthful and happy life for the women in this country effortless and enjoyable, and I couldn't have a better ally for my Carb Swap message.

To Jacqui Stafford, the Executive Style Director of *Shape* magazine, who has taught me so much about the deeper side of beauty and style—your insights into the power of confidence have truly helped make my message stronger.

To Jared Davis, the member of my team who has been supporting me and my mission longer than anyone else—your commitment and artistic talent make what I do not only possible, but downright beautiful and inspiring. Not only are you an amazing artist, but I truly consider you to be one of my very best friends. I cannot thank you enough for all the ways in which you have supported not only my work, but my person. Thank you.

To Oliver Stephenson, the only person I've ever been able to trust with managing our mission so effectively—your attention to detail, loyalty, and character not only inspire me but make my work possible and my life enjoyable. You are literally managing the Carb Swap revolution, and our entire team is grateful for your leadership. Without you, this puzzle would have remained in pieces, and the future of our entire team is brighter for the talents you bring to the table. Thank you, buddy.

To Michelle McGowen and Kimberly Barry, the two women who keep our entire team grounded—both of you show a tremendous passion for the mission, and bring a nurturing energy that our team couldn't function without. The hard work and positivity you bring to the table remind us of our mission each and every day.

To Louise Hay, Reid Tracy, Stacey Smith, and the incredible support team at Hay House—a huge and heartfelt thanks! The mix of passion and professionalism at Hay House is astounding, and the level of quality you bring to my work cannot be overstated.

Thank you to Pearl Hodges for your amazing illustrations that added such an engaging element to this book, to Sarah Dubina for your methodical assistance with the massive amount of research that went into this project, to Robbie McMillin for your invaluable editorial contributions, and to Kathy Valentine for your editor's eye. I'd also like to thank Christy Stevenson and Marco Montano for the style and aesthetic touch they brought to the clients in this book.

I'm also incredibly grateful to my amazing mentors in health and nutrition. To Dr. Christiane Northrup—connecting with you has been truly eye-opening. I learned so much from you about the special consequences of sugar for women that it literally shaped my mission in life. Being invited to participate in your PBS special and being honored by your Foreword to this book were a dream come true.

To Dr. Andrew Weil—your continued support over the years has meant so much. More than any other M.D. in the public eye, your pursuit of a more integrative approach to health is exactly the message our society needs in these dire times.

To Mark Sisson—you are such a personal inspiration for me, and I'm incredibly grateful for the point of view and knowledge you have brought to the table in our partnership. I greatly look forward to all our future collaborations.

Thank you to my entire circle of invaluable health experts: Dr. Mehmet Oz, Dr. David Katz, Dr. James Novak, Dr. Terry Grossman, Dr. Ray Kurzweil, Dr. Nicholas Perricone, and Gary Taubes. I'm fortunate to have such renowned experts as mentors and friends.

A very special thanks to my friends and partners in the media, who have been so vital in spreading this critical message: Rachael Ray, Abra Potkin, Janet Annino, John Redmann, Terence Noonan, Ginnie Roeglin, Anita Thompson, David Fuller, Tim

Talevish, Maggie Jacqua, Beth Weissman, Scott Eason, Al Roker, Mark Victor, Bill Getty, Joy Behar, Thomas Walter, Priscilla Totten, Terry Wood, Maggie Barnes, Loren Nancarrow, Leslie Marcus, and Richard Heller.

To Denise Vivaldo and Jon Edwards—thank you for adding such beautiful and delicious food to this project.

To my amazing clients—you inspired me to believe that each and every person has the innate ability to seize the day and reach for the life of his or her dreams. A very special thanks to Amber Allen-Sauer, who didn't stop at just helping herself—your giving nature and passion for spreading this message is exactly the kind of enthusiasm that drives positive change in our world.

I'd also like to thank my good friends for their support this past year: Lisa Sharkey, Joe Boleware, Jeff Craig, Bo Bortner, Rich Segal, Lauri Stock, Dr. Bob Hirsch, Suze Orman, Bob Wietrak, Mary-Ellen Keating, Richard Galanti, Debbie Ford, Pennie Ianniciello, Mike Koenings, Jay Robb, Frank Kern, Chris Hendrickson, Anthony Robbins, Eben Pagan, Elliot Bisnow, Suzanne Somers, and Wayne Dyer.

Finally, I am tremendously grateful to my dearest friend, Heather Cruise, a beautiful and understanding woman with whom I share two amazing sons. Thank you for all of your love, support, and belief for so many years. The best is yet to come. I love you very much, forever.

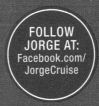

About the Author

JORGE CRUISE is the #1 *New York Times* best-selling author of over 20 diet and fitness books in over 16 languages, including *8 Minutes in the Morning*, *The Belly Fat Cure*, *The 100*, and *Happy Hormones, Slim Belly*. He is a contributor to *The Dr. Oz Show*, *Steve Harvey*, *Good Morning America,* the *Today* show, the *Rachael Ray Show*, *Huffington Post*, *First for Women* magazine, and the *Costco Connection*.

Jorge received his bachelor's degree from the University of California, San Diego (UCSD); and has fitness credentials from the Cooper Institute for Aerobics Research, the American College of Sports Medicine (ACSM), and the American Council on Exercise (ACE).

To find out more about Jorge, visit **JorgeCruise.com**

We hope you enjoyed this Hay House book. If you'd like to receive our online catalog featuring additional information on Hay House books and products, or if you'd like to find out more about the Hay Foundation, please contact:

Hay House, Inc.,
P.O. Box 5100, Carlsbad, CA 92018-5100

(760) 431-7695 or (800) 654-5126
(760) 431-6948 (fax) or (800) 650-5115 (fax)
www.hayhouse.com® • www.hayfoundation.org

• • •

Published and distributed in Australia by:
Hay House Australia Pty. Ltd., 18/36 Ralph St., Alexandria NSW 2015 •
Phone: 612-9669-4299 • *Fax:* 612-9669-4144 • www.hayhouse.com.au

Published and distributed in the United Kingdom by:
Hay House UK, Ltd., Astley House, 33 Notting Hill Gate, London W11 3JQ
Phone: 44-20-3675-2450 • *Fax:* 44-20-3675-2451 • www.hayhouse.co.uk

Published and distributed in the Republic of South Africa by:
Hay House SA (Pty), Ltd., P.O. Box 990, Witkoppen 2068 • *Phone/Fax:* 27-11-467-8904 •
www.hayhouse.co.za

Published in India by:
Hay House Publishers India, Muskaan Complex, Plot No. 3, B-2, Vasant Kunj, New Delhi 110 070 •
Phone: 91-11-4176-1620 • *Fax:* 91-11-4176-1630 • www.hayhouse.co.in

Distributed in Canada by:
Raincoast Books, 2440 Viking Way, Richmond, B.C. V6V 1N2
Phone: 1-800-663-5714 • *Fax:* 1-800-565-3770 • www.raincoast.com

• • •

Take Your Soul on a Vacation

Visit **www.HealYourLife.com**® to regroup, recharge, and reconnect
with your own magnificence. Featuring blogs, mind-body-spirit news,
and life-changing wisdom from Louise Hay and friends.

Visit **www.HealYourLife.com** today!

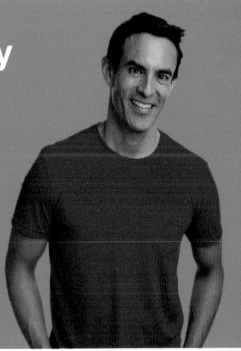

As a parent and someone whose mission is focused on improving the health of future generations, I am proud to support the work of President Bill Clinton and his Alliance for a Healthier Generation.

Working together with the American Heart Association, the Alliance for a Healthier Generation works with more than 10,000 schools, helping them increase physical activity and offering healthy food and beverage options. I highly recommend that you sign your school up for this program at: **www.HealthierGeneration.org.**

Also working together with the Alliance, the Michael & Susan Dell Foundation has helped create a free resource for parents that offers tips on tough topics like getting kids to eat more vegetables. The website, **www.BeWellBook.org**, is a must for all parents who wish to see their children develop healthy habits that last a lifetime.

Check out their amazing work and pledge your support to this incredibly worthwhile cause!